Atlas of Emergency Ultrasound

Atlas of Emergency Ultrasound

Edited by

John Christian Fox
University of California, Irvine School of Medicine, CA, USA

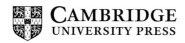

CAMBRIDGE
UNIVERSITY PRESS

CAMBRIDGE UNIVERSITY PRESS

Cambridge, New York, Melbourne, Madrid, Cape Town,
Singapore, São Paulo, Delhi, Tokyo, Mexico City

Cambridge University Press
The Edinburgh Building, Cambridge CB2 8RU, UK

Published in the United States of America by
Cambridge University Press, New York

www.cambridge.org
Information on this title: www.cambridge.org/9780521191685

First published 2011

Printed in the United Kingdom at the University Press, Cambridge

A catalog record for this publication is available from the British Library

Library of Congress Cataloging-in-Publication Data

Atlas of emergency ultrasound / edited by John Christian Fox.
    p. ; cm.
  Includes index.
  ISBN 978-0-521-19168-5 (hbk.)
    1. Diagnostic ultrasonic imaging–Atlases.   2. Emergency medicine–
Diagnosis–Atlases.   I. Fox, J. Christian.
    [DNLM: 1. Ultrasonography–Atlases.   2. Emergency Treatment–
Atlases.   WN 17]
    RC78.7.U4A85 2011
    616.07′543–dc22

                                                                    2011008590

ISBN 978-0-521-19168-5 Hardback

**WN
17
A881
2011**

Contents

List of contributors vi

Preface vii

1. **Focused assessment of sonography in trauma** 1
   Patricia Fermin and John Christian Fox

2. **Ocular ultrasound** 19
   George Mittendorf and John Christian Fox

3. **Cardiac ultrasound** 26
   Shane Summers

4. **Ultrasound of the lung** 35
   Justin Davis and Seric Cusick

5. **Right upper quadrant ultrasonography** 58
   Daniel Gromis and John Christian Fox

6. **Intestinal ultrasound** 77
   Warren Wiechmann and Chase Warren

7. **Pelvic ultrasound** 88
   Cindy Chau and John Christian Fox

8. **Genitourinary ultrasound** 103
   Christina Umber and John Christian Fox

9. **Musculoskeletal ultrasound** 133
   Deborah Shipley Kane and Jennifer McBride

10. **Pediatric ultrasound** 141
    Stephanie Doniger and George Mittendorf

11. **Ultrasound-guided procedures** 158
    Eric J. Chin

12. **Arterial ultrasound** 175
    Sharis Simonian and John Christian Fox

13. **Venous ultrasound** 185
    Kevin Burns and John Christian Fox

Index 191

Contributors

Kevin Burns
New York University School of Medicine, New York,
New York, USA

Cindy Chau, MD
Resident, OB/GYN, University of California, Irvine
Medical Center, Orange, California, USA

Eric J. Chin, MD, RDMS, MAJ, USA, MC
Associate Program Director, Emergency Ultrasound
Fellowship, Staff Emergency Physician, Brooke Army
Medical Center, San Antonio Uniformed Services
Health Education Consortium,
San Antonio, Texas, USA

Seric Cusick, MD, RDMS
Department of Emergency Medicine,
Hoag Hospital, Newport Beach, California, USA

Justin Davis
Kaiser Oakland Medical Center,
Oakland, California, USA

Stephanie Doniger, MD, RDMS
Director of Emergency Ultrasound, Children's
Hospital and Research Center Oakland, Oakland,
California, USA

Patricia Fermin, MD
Resident, Emergency Medicine,
Harbor-UCLA Medical Center, Los Angeles,
California, USA

John Christian Fox, MD, Clinical RDMS
Professor of Emergency Medicine, Director of
Instructional Ultrasound, University of California,
Irvine Medical Center, Orange, California, USA

Daniel Gromis, MD
Resident, Emergency Medicine, Advocate Christ
Hospital and Medical Center, Chicago, Illinois, USA

Jennifer McBride, MD
Resident, Emergency Medicine,
Georgetown University, Washington, DC,
USA

George Mittendorf, MD
Resident, Emergency Medicine,
UCSF – Fresno, Fresno, California,
USA

Deborah Shipley Kane, MD, RDMS
Clinical Instructor, Ultrasound Director,
Washington University of St. Louis,
St. Louis, Missouri, USA

Sharis Simonian, MD
Resident, Emergency Medicine,
University of California, Irvine, Orange,
California, USA

Shane Summers, MD, RDMS
Program Director, Emergency Ultrasound
Fellowship, Assistant Professor of Military and
Emergency Medicine,
San Antonio Uniformed Services Health Education
Consortium, San Antonio, Texas,
USA

Christina Umber, MD
Resident, Emergency Medicine,
UCSF – Fresno, Fresno,
California, USA

Chase Warren
University of California, Irvine, Orange,
California, USA

Warren Wiechmann, MD, RDMS
Assistant Professor of Emergency Medicine,
UCSF – Fresno, Fresno, California,
USA

Preface

When a physician examines a patient at the bedside using the physical exam alone they are forced to rely on their "mind's eye" to *imagine* what organs or tissue below the skin that could be the culprit of their patient's ailment. With the advent of portable bedside ultrasound, physicians are now able to *image* the organs and tissue directly at the point-of-care, creating an immediate impact on patient care. Harnessing this technology transforms the doctor–patient relationship from the time of Hippocrates to the modern day. Physician-performed imaging results in greater clinical self-reliance, reducing unnecessary CT scans, thereby causing less radiation exposure.

The *Atlas of Emergency Ultrasound* is designed to give the busy practicing clinician a reference tool of positives. Each organ is represented with common and not so common pathological entities one encounters when practicing emergency ultrasound. This pathology is clearly outlined by line-art, with detailed captions drawing the reader to salient points. This is *not* meant to be an exhaustive didactic reference, or even an introduction to obtaining ultrasound windows. This book picks up where introductory coursework ends. There already exist plenty of references designed to teach the basics of image acquisition and ultrasound physics. This book assumes the reader has already begun to incorporate ultrasound into practice, and is now ready to take those skills further by focusing on pathology.

While the focus is on *emergency* ultrasound, there are other specialties that would likely benefit from the pathology found in this text. Physicians who practice primary care will likely find many relevant images to learn from especially with regards to the gallbladder, pelvis, and vasculature, while physicians in the ICU setting will find the cardiac, DVT, and lung chapters of particular interest. Furthermore, surgeons looking for pathology related to the hepato-biliary system, soft tissue, and vasculature will find information relevant to their practice. Finally, as medical students are expected to perform more and more ultrasound at the bedside of their patients on rotations in the emergency department, the ICU, surgery, and Obst/Gyn, they too will find helpful images to help them perform well on these clerkships.

Ultimately, Hippocrates would be proud of the physician who can utilize any simple bedside tool to elaborate on the physical exam, but only if that tool would result in "first do no harm."

Chapter 1

Focused assessment of sonography in trauma

Patricia Fermin and John Christian Fox

Epicardial fat pad

When imaging the heart, careful attention must be made in identifying any surrounding fluid. The presence of epicardial fat should be ruled out to have a clear determination of the presence of fluid.

Hemopericardium

An examination of the heart is crucial during trauma to the chest, such as a stabbing, gunshot wound, or motor vehicle collision. The identification of blood surrounding the heart is critical in order to prevent or

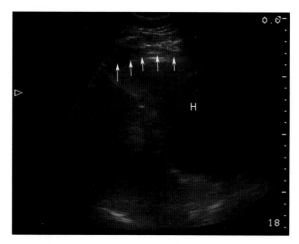

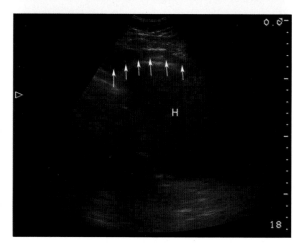

Epicardial fat pad: In this subxiphoid view, the four chambers of the heart (H) are difficult to visualize. However, a layer of fat (arrows) surrounding the heart may be seen. It is important to distinguish epicardial fat from hemopericardium, which is more echolucent.

Atlas of Emergency Ultrasound, ed. John Christian Fox. Published by Cambridge University Press. © J.C. Fox 2011.

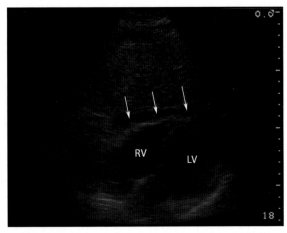

Hemopericardium: In this subxiphoid view, blood (arrows) surrounding the heart is found in a patient stabbed through the chest. There is a clear view of the echolucent space between the visceral and parietal pericardium and the right ventricle (RV) and left ventricle (LV).

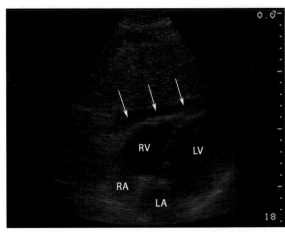

Hemopericardium: In this subxiphoid view, blood (arrows) surrounding the heart is found in a patient stabbed through the chest. There is a clear view of the echolucent space between the visceral and parietal pericardium and the right ventricle (RV), left ventricle (LV), right atrium (RA), and left atrium (LA).

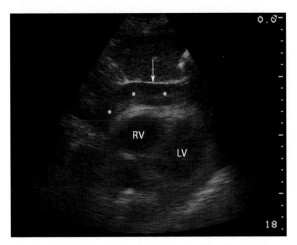

Hemopericardium: In this subxiphoid view, blood (asterisks) surrounding the heart is found in a patient stabbed through the chest. There is a clear view of the echolucent space between the visceral and parietal pericardium and the right ventricle (RV) and left ventricle (LV). The arrow refers to the anterior pericardium.

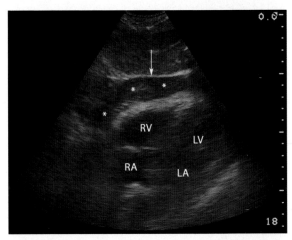

Hemopericardium: In this subxiphoid view, blood (asterisks) surrounding the heart is found in a patient stabbed through the chest. There is a clear view of the echolucent space between the visceral and parietal pericardium and the right ventricle (RV), left ventricle (LV), right atrium (RA), and left atrium (LA). The arrow refers to the anterior pericardium.

treat cardiac tamponade. The contractility of the heart will also assist in determining the severity of the hemopericardium.

Left chest view

The view of the left chest is additionally essential with trauma to the chest, such as in a stabbing, gunshot wound, or motor vehicle collision. The diaphragm is a significant marker, which will have the fluid superior to it. Fluid found in this area reveals a traumatic hemothorax.

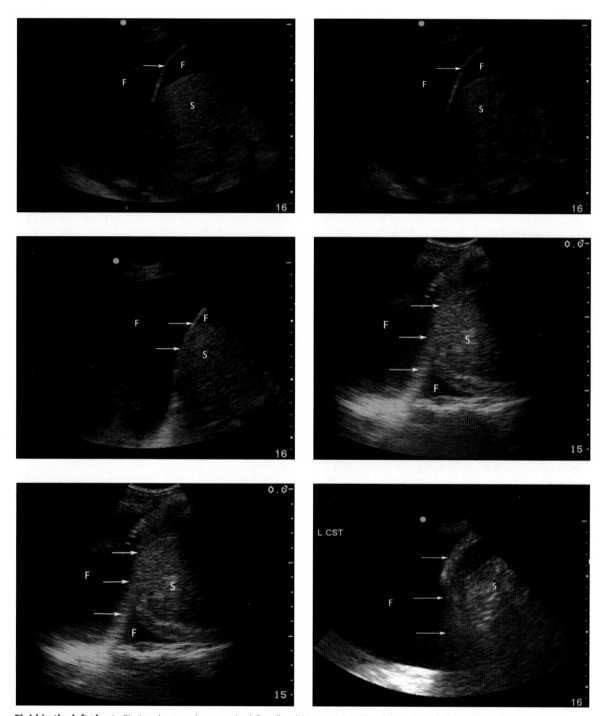

Fluid in the left chest: Placing the transducer on the left axillary line superior to the rib margin with the indicator facing up, reveals fluid (F) in the patient's left chest. The spleen (S) and diaphragm (arrows) are clearly visualized. This view is useful when there is trauma to the chest, such as in a motor vehicle collision, stabbing, or gunshot wound.

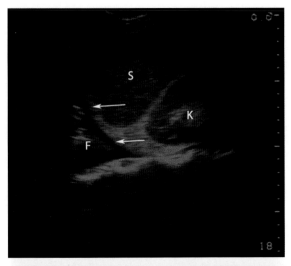

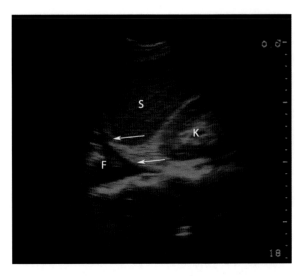

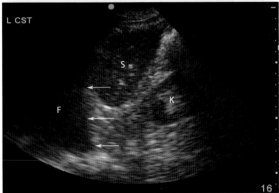

Fluid in the left chest: Placing the transducer on the left axillary line superior to the rib margin with the indicator facing up, reveals fluid (F) in the patient's left chest. The spleen (S), kidney (K), and diaphragm (arrows) are clearly visualized. This view is useful when there is a trauma to the chest, such as in a motor vehicle collision, stabbing, or gunshot wound.

Morrison's pouch

The examination of the Morrison's pouch, the recess between the liver and kidney is crucial during trauma to the abdomen or pelvis. Damage to internal organs and blood vessels will result in fluid settling in this area primarily. A clear view of the liver and kidney should be obtained, which normally would not present with fluid in between.

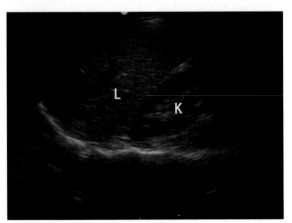

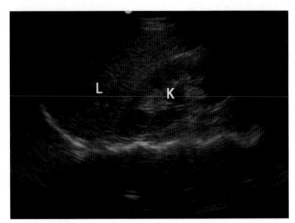

Normal view of Morrison's pouch: In this normal view of the Morrison's pouch, the recess between the liver and kidney, the transducer is placed in the right axillary line at the rib margin with the indicator facing up. There is a clear view of the liver (L) and kidney (K) with no presence of fluid.

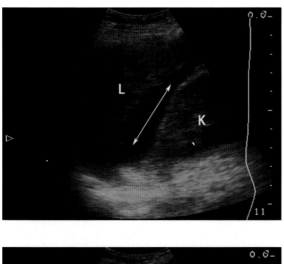

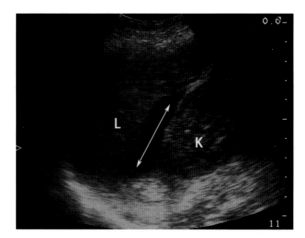

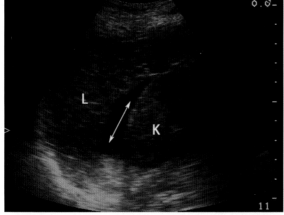

Fluid in Morrison's pouch: In this view, there is remarkable free fluid (double arrow) in Morrison's pouch, between the liver (L) and kidney (K). This is valuable during blunt trauma to the abdomen or pelvis causing damage to internal organs and blood vessels, with fluid settling in this area.

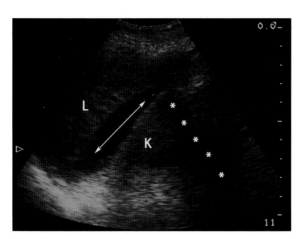

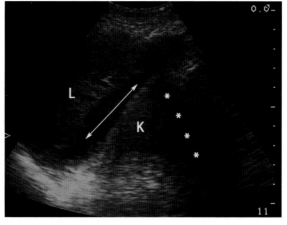

Fluid in Morrison's pouch: In this view, there is remarkable free fluid (double arrow) in Morrison's pouch, between the liver (L) and kidney (K). This is valuable during blunt trauma to the abdomen or pelvis causing damage to internal organs and blood vessels, with fluid settling in this area. Keep in mind that rib shadow (asterisk) may obstruct the view.

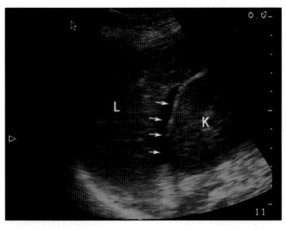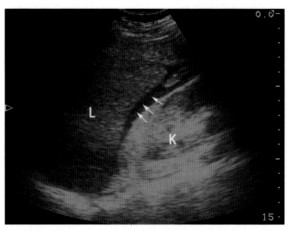

Fluid in Morrison's pouch: In this view, there is remarkable free fluid (arrows) in Morrison's pouch, between the liver (L) and kidney (K). This is valuable during blunt trauma to the abdomen or pelvis causing damage to internal organs and blood vessels, with fluid settling in this area.

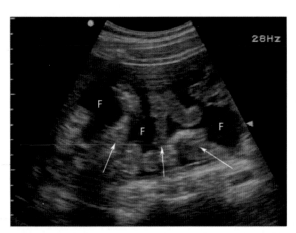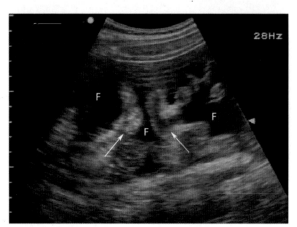

Fluid around loops of bowel: In this view, the transducer is placed on the lower abdomen of the patient. There is a clear view of free fluid (F) around the loops of bowel (arrows).

Pelvis

Examining the lower abdomen of a patient after a trauma may reveal free fluid around bowel. This is a sign that major injury has occurred in the abdomen or pelvis.

Pericardial clot

While examining the heart, a pericardial clot may be visualized instead of newly escaped blood. This reveals that the trauma has occurred for a significant period and careful examination of heart activity should be performed.

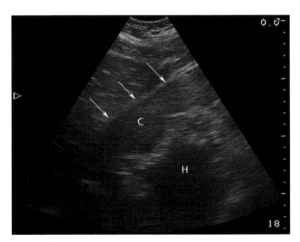 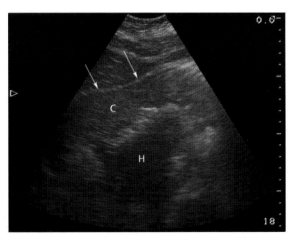

Pericardial clot: This subxiphoid view was obtained on a patient with a gunshot wound to the chest. The chambers of the heart (H) are not clearly visualized; however, an echodense clot (C) between the visceral and parietal pericardium (arrows) may be seen.

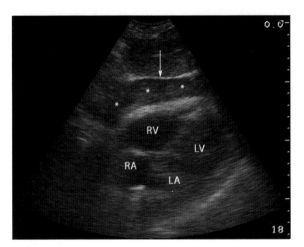 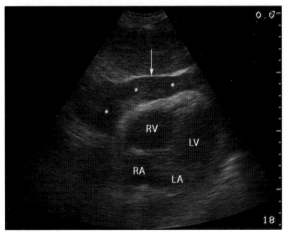

Pericardial clot: This subxiphoid view was obtained on a patient with a gunshot wound to the chest. All four chambers of the heart are clearly visualized – the right ventricle (RV), left ventricle (LV), right atrium (RA) and the left atrium (LA). Additionally, an echodense clot (asterisk) between the visceral and parietal pericardium (arrow) may be seen.

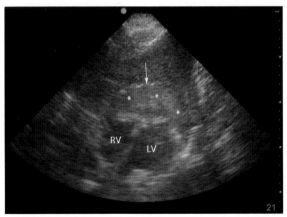 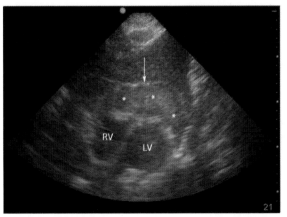

Pericardial clot: This subxiphoid view was obtained on a patient with a gunshot wound to the chest. The right ventricle (RV) and left ventricle (LV) of the heart are clearly visualized. Additionally, an echodense clot (asterisks) between the visceral and parietal pericardium (arrow) may be seen.

Perinephric fat

While visualizing Morrison's pouch and the spleno-renal recess, careful consideration of perinephric fat should be obtained. This should not be mistaken for free fluid, which has contrasting echogenicities.

Right chest

The view of the right chest is essential as well when performing an exam on the left side with trauma to the chest. The diaphragm is a significant marker, which will have the fluid superior and the liver inferior to it. Fluid found in this area reveals a traumatic hemothorax.

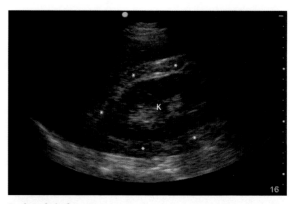

Perinephric fat: This view reveals fat (asterisks) surrounding the kidney (K), which should not be mistaken for free fluid, with its increased echogenicity.

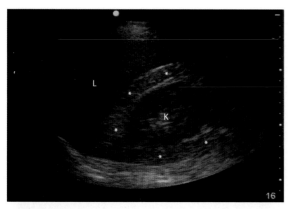

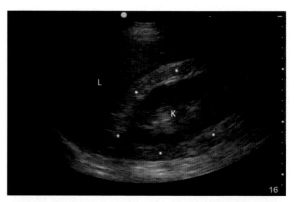

Perinephric fat: This view reveals fat (asterisks) surrounding the kidney (K) and a clear view of the adjacent liver (L). This should not be mistaken for free fluid, with its increased echogenicity.

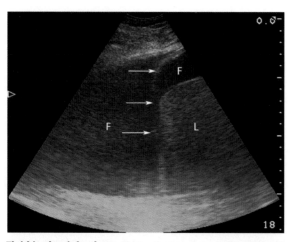

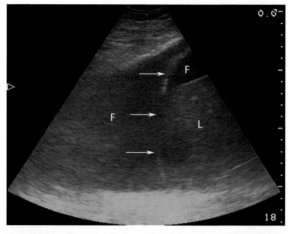

Fluid in the right chest: Placing the transducer on the right axillary line, superior to the rib with the indicator facing up reveals fluid (F) in the patient's right chest. This fluid is bordered by the diaphragm (arrows) below and with a clear view of the liver (L). This view is also useful when there is trauma to the chest, such as in a motor vehicle collision, stabbing, or gunshot wound.

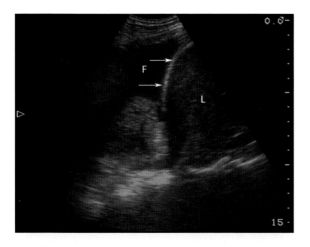

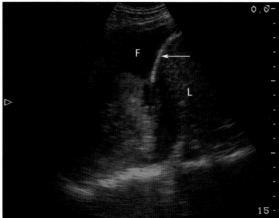

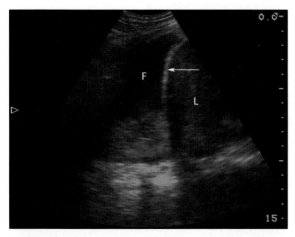

Fluid in the right chest: *(cont.)*

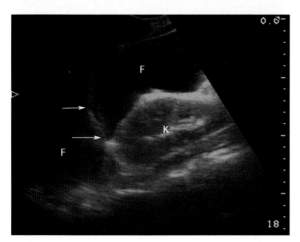

Fluid in the right chest: Placing the transducer on the right axillary line, superior to the rib with the indicator facing up reveals fluid (F) in the patient's right chest. This fluid is bordered by the diaphragm (arrows) below and with a clear view of the kidney (K). This view is also useful when there is trauma to the chest, such as in a motor vehicle collision, stabbing, or gunshot wound.

Splenorenal view

The examination of the splenorenal recess is additionally crucial during trauma to the abdomen or pelvis. Damage to internal organs and blood vessels will result in fluid settling in this area primarily. A clear view of the spleen and kidney should be obtained, which normally would not present with fluid in between. Fluid found in the stomach which is superior to the spleen and kidney should not be mistaken for fluid in the chest, which is adjacent to the diaphragm.

9

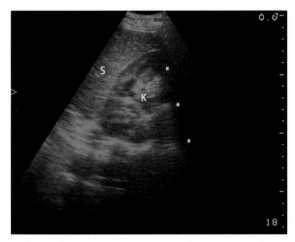

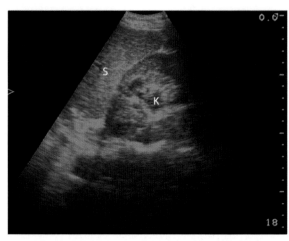

Normal splenorenal view: In this normal view, there is no fluid present in the recess between the spleen (S) and kidney (K). The transducer is placed in the left axillary line at the rib margin with the indicator facing up. Keep in mind that rib shadow (asterisks) may obstruct the view.

Normal splenorenal view: In this normal view, there is no fluid present in the recess between the spleen (S) and kidney (K). The transducer is placed in the left axillary line at the rib margin with the indicator facing up.

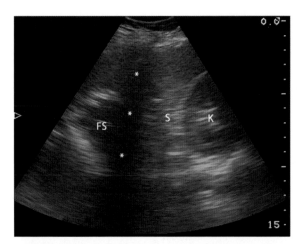

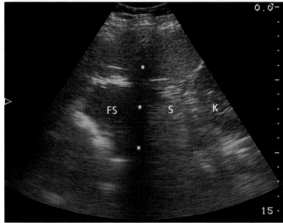

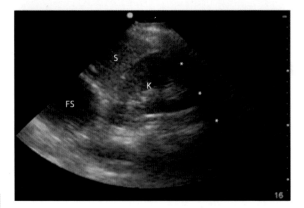

Fluid in the stomach with the splenorenal view: In this view of the splenorenal recess, the stomach which is superior to the spleen (S) and kidney (K) is found to have fluid (FS). This should not be mistaken for fluid in the chest, which is adjacent to the diaphragm. Keep in mind that rib shadow (asterisks) may obstruct the view.

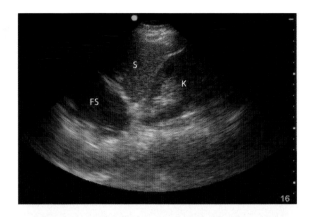

Fluid in the stomach with the splenorenal view: In this view of the splenorenal recess, the stomach which is superior to the spleen (S) and kidney (K) is found to have fluid (FS). This should not be mistaken for fluid in the chest, which is adjacent to the diaphragm.

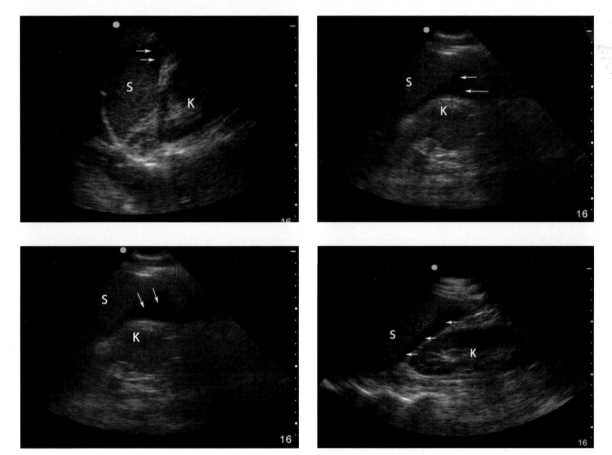

Fluid in the splenorenal recess: In this view, there is remarkable free fluid (F) between the spleen (S) and kidney (K). This view is also valuable during blunt trauma to the abdomen or pelvis causing damage to internal organs and blood vessels, with fluid settling in this area.

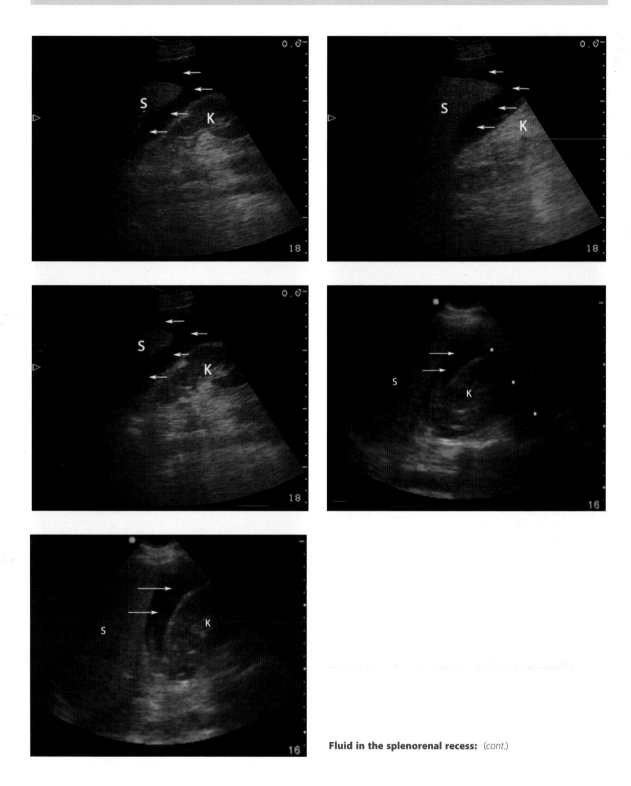

Fluid in the splenorenal recess: (*cont.*)

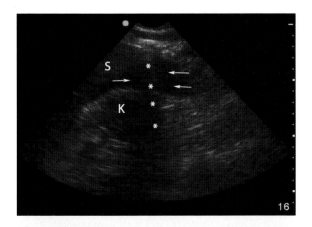

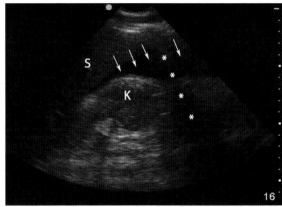

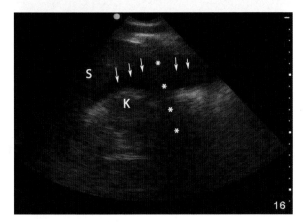

Fluid in the splenorenal recess: In this view, there is remarkable free fluid (F) between the spleen (S) and kidney (K). This view is also valuable during blunt trauma to the abdomen or pelvis causing damage to internal organs and blood vessels, with fluid settling in this area. Keep in mind that rib shadow (asterisks) may obstruct the view.

Suprapubic view

An examination of the suprapubic area is essential for suspected damage to the pelvic region especially with blunt trauma such as in a motor vehicle collision. The bladder should be clearly visualized with the presence of the uterus more posterior depending on the patient.

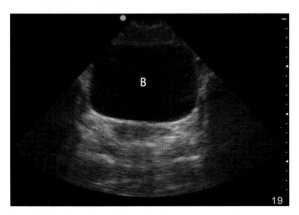

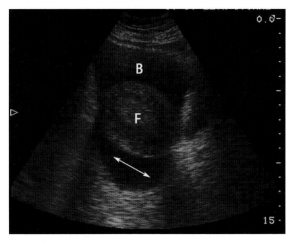

Normal suprapubic view: In this suprapubic view, the echolucent bladder (B) is clearly visualized without any surrounding fluid. The transducer is placed midline just superior to the pubic symphysis with indicator to patient's right.

Fluid in suprapubic region: In this suprapubic view of a female patient, fluid (double arrow) is visualized surrounding the uterus possessing a fibroid (F) with the bladder (B) anterior to it. This view is important during trauma with suspected damage to the pelvic region.

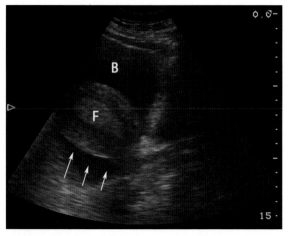 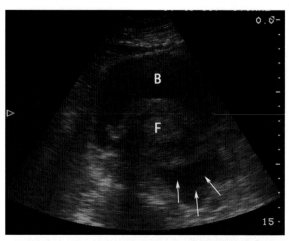

Fluid in suprapubic region: In this suprapubic view of a female patient, fluid (arrows) is visualized surrounding the uterus possessing a fibroid (F) with the bladder (B) anterior to it. This view is important during trauma with suspected damage to the pelvic region.

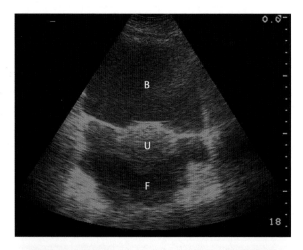

Fluid in a female suprapubic region: In this suprapubic view of a female patient, fluid (F) is visualized surrounding the uterus (U) with the bladder (B) anterior to it. This view is important during trauma with suspected damage to the pelvic region.

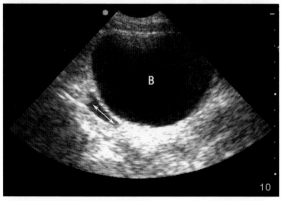 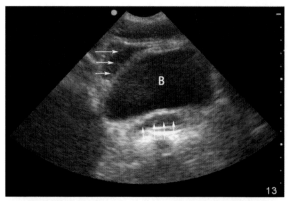

Fluid in male suprapubic region: In this suprapubic view of a male patient, fluid (arrows) is visualized surrounding the bladder (B). This view is important during trauma with suspected damage to the pelvic region.

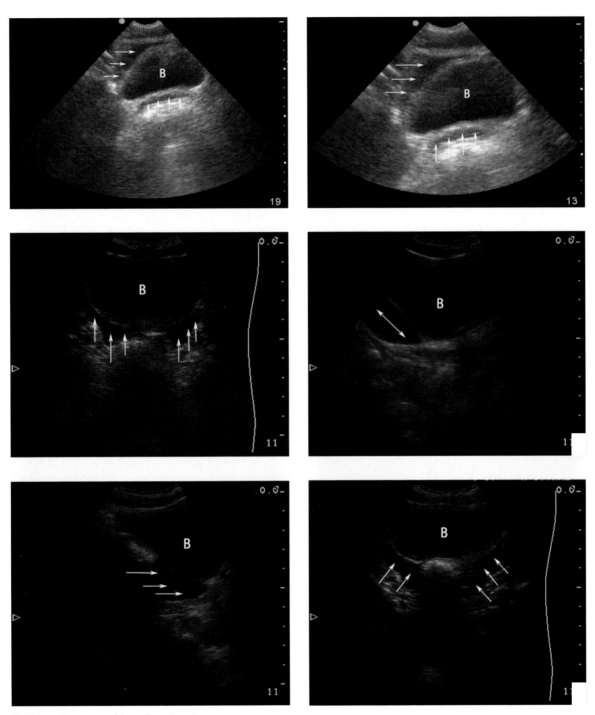

Fluid in male suprapubic region: (*cont.*)

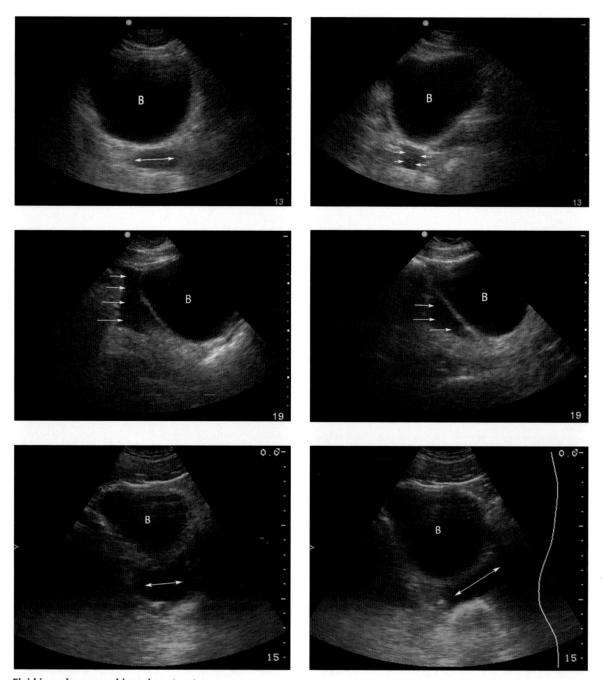

Fluid in male suprapubic region: *(cont.)*

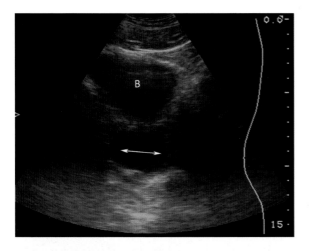

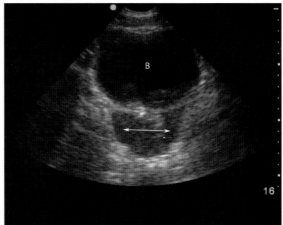

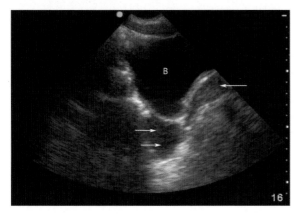

Fluid in male suprapubic region: (*cont.*)

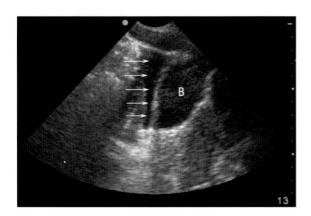

Fluid in male suprapubic region with cross-sectional view: In this suprapubic view of a male patient, fluid (arrows) is visualized surrounding the bladder (B) seen in the cross-sectional view.

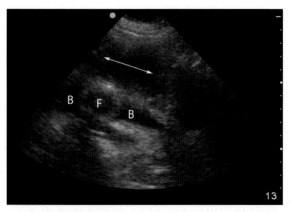 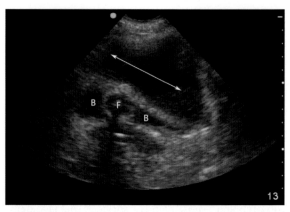

Fluid in male suprapubic region: In this suprapubic view of a male patient, fluid (arrow) is visualized surrounding the collapsed bladder (B) due to an apparent Foley catheter (F). This view is important during trauma with suspected damage to the pelvic region.

Chapter 2

Ocular ultrasound

George Mittendorf and John Christian Fox

Damaged globe

Ultrasound can expedite the identification of a globe rupture and subsequently surgical management. Important characteristics to look for include overall shape and size of the globe, asymmetry, and a collapsed anterior chamber.

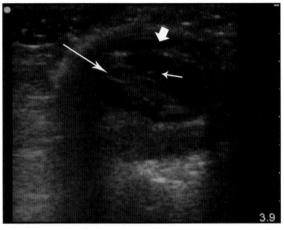

Gunshot wound to right eye: Traumatic path of projectile (long arrow), posterior aspect of lens (short arrow), anterior chamber (fat arrow).

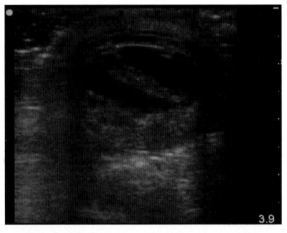

Gunshot wound: Gunshot wound to right eye.

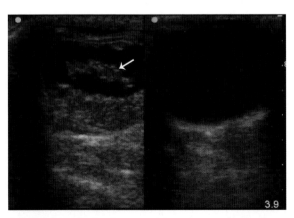

Gunshot wound: Gunshot wound through eye and patient's unaffected eye.

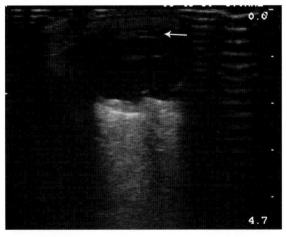

Ruptured globe: Ruptured globe demonstrating decreased size, asymmetric shape, and collapsed anterior chamber (arrow).

Atlas of Emergency Ultrasound, ed. John Christian Fox. Published by Cambridge University Press. © J.C. Fox 2011.

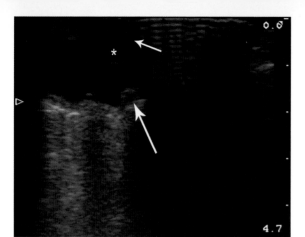

Ruptured globe: Ruptured globe, buckling sclera (long arrow), collapsed anterior chamber (short arrow), lens (*).

Optic nerve

The optic nerve has recently become an increasingly important aspect to examine because of its relationship with elevated intracranial pressure. The optic nerve can be easily found by looking posterior to the globe for a hypoechoic region that runs perpendicular to the probe's footprint.

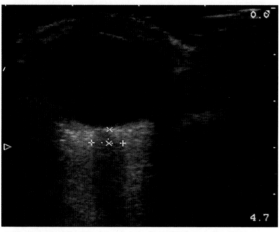

Measurement of the optic nerve sheath diameter: Measurement of the optic nerve sheath diameter (horizontal measurement) 3 mm proximal to the optic disc (vertical measurement). Optic nerve sheath diameter is greater than 5 mm, indicating elevated intracranial pressure.

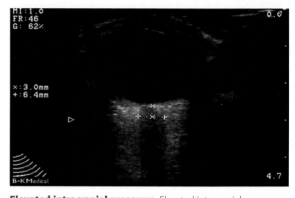

Elevated intracranial pressure: Elevated intracranial pressure as evidenced by an optic nerve sheath diameter greater than 5 mm (+'s). Note the diameter is measured 3 mm posterior to the globe, (x's) which allows measurement within an area of better contrast.

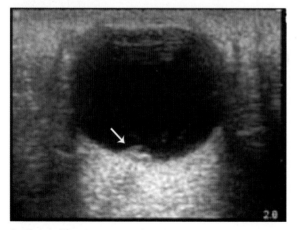

Optic neuritis: Optic neuritis (arrow).

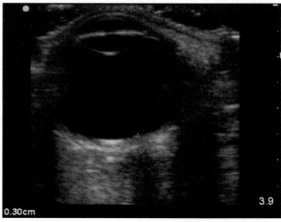

Where to measure optic disc nerve sheath: Measure 3 mm posterior to globe.

Retinal detachments

Ultrasound is an effective way of quickly diagnosing a retinal detachment. The detached retina can be seen as a mobile and fluid hyperechoic line that undulates especially with movement of the eye. Furthermore one can visualize it tethered to the posterior aspect of the eye at the optic disc.

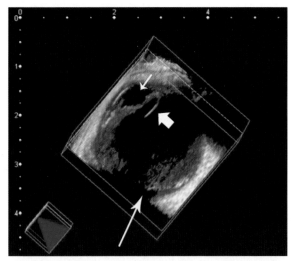

Retinal detachment: 3D reconstruction of retinal detachment (skinny arrow). Anterior chamber (small arrow), posterior surface of lens (fat arrow).

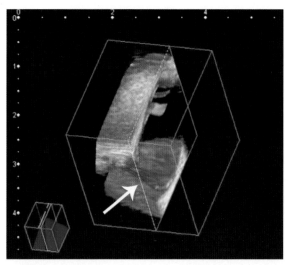

Retinal detachment: Retinal detachment (arrow).

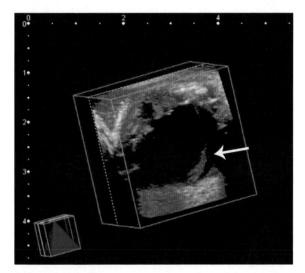

Retinal detachment: 3D reconstruction of retinal detachment.

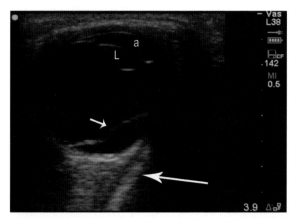

Retinal detachment: Retinal detachment (small arrow), anterior chamber (a), lens (L), lateral rectus muscle (long arrow).

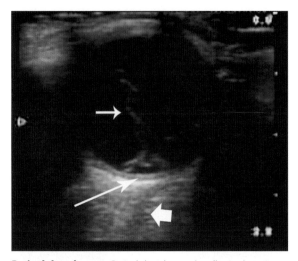

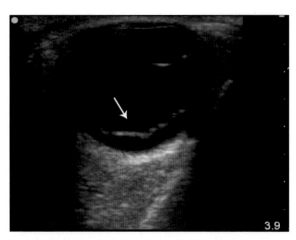

Retinal detachment: Retinal detachment (small arrow), optic nerve (fat arrow), optic disc (long arrow).

Retinal detachment: Retinal detachment (arrow).

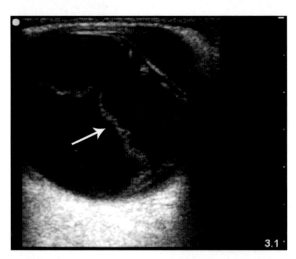

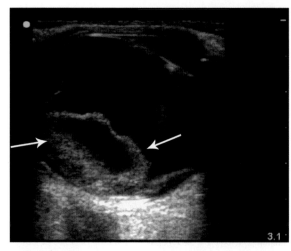

Retinal detachment: Retinal detachment (arrow).

Retinal detachment: Retinal detachment (arrows).

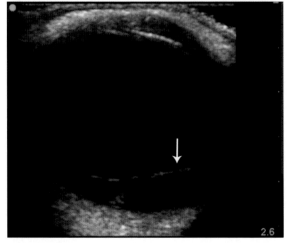

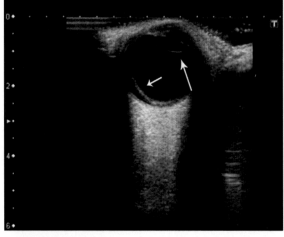

Retinal detachment: Retinal detachment (arrow).

Retinal detachment: Retinal detachment (small arrow). Lens (large arrow).

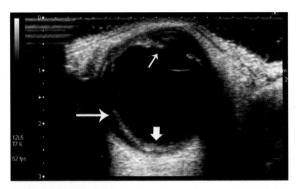

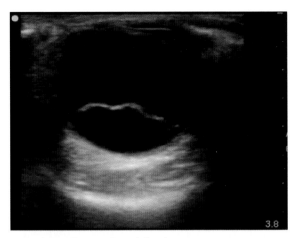

Retinal detachment: Retinal detachment (large arrow), iris (small arrow), optic disc (fat arrow).

Retinal detachment: Retinal detachment.

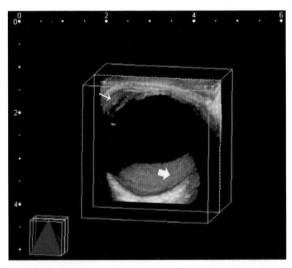

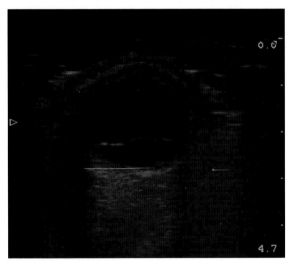

Retinal detachment: 3D reconstruction of normal eye. Anterior chamber (small arrow), retina (fat arrow).

Retinal detachment: Retinal detachment.

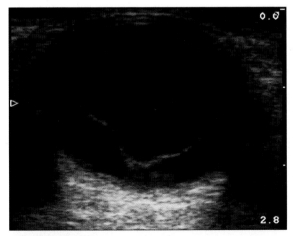

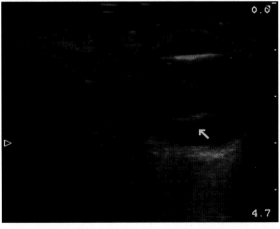

Retinal detachment: Retinal detachment.

Retinal detachment: Retinal detachment (arrow).

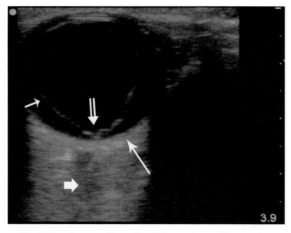

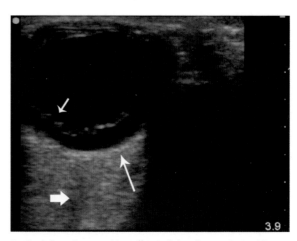

Retinal detachment: Mac-off retinal detachment. Retina (short arrow), optic nerve (fat arrow), macula (long arrow), tether point of retina to optic disc (double arrow).

Retinal detachment: Mac-off retinal detachment. Retina (short arrow), macula (long arrow), optic nerve (fat arrow).

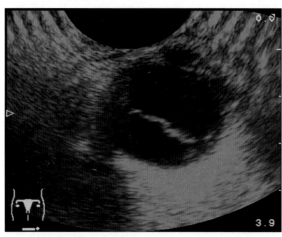

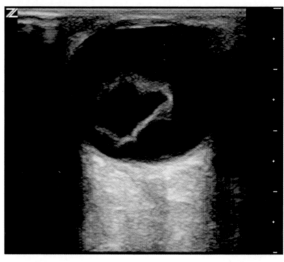

Retinal detachment: Retinal detachment as evidenced with endovaginal probe.

Retinal detachment: Large retinal detachment. View is capturing the rim around a protruding portion of retina.

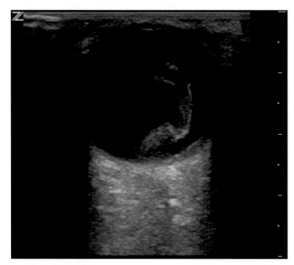

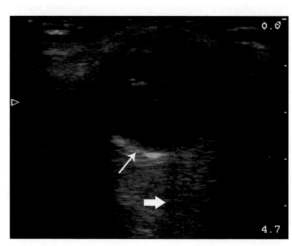

Retinal detachment: Large retinal detachment.

Retinal detachment: Mac-off retinal detachment. Optic nerve (fat arrow), macula (skinny arrow).

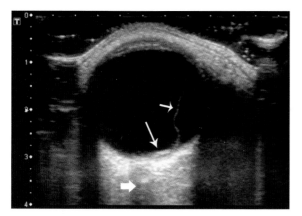

Retinal detachment: Mac-on retinal detachment. Optic nerve (fat arrow), macula (long arrow), detached retina (short arrow).

Vitreous

Although sometimes confused with retinal detachments, a vitreous hemorrhage can be identified as a swirling, slightly hyperechoic focus in the posterior globe.

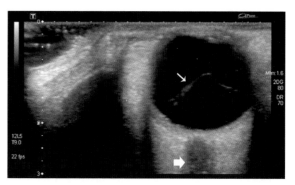

Vitreous detachment: Detached vitreous (short arrow), optic nerve (fat arrow).

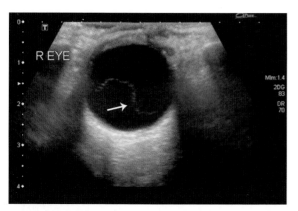

Detached vitreous body: Detached vitreous body that looks like a retinal detachment.

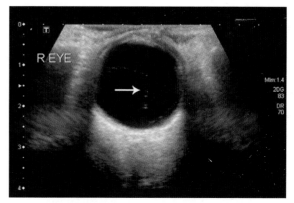

Detached vitreous body: Another detached vitreous body (arrow) that looks like a retinal detachment.

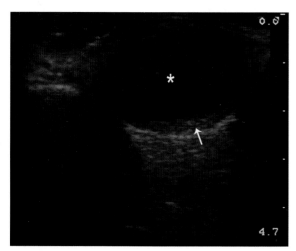

Vitreous hemorrhage: Vitreous hemorrhage (arrow), vitreous body (*).

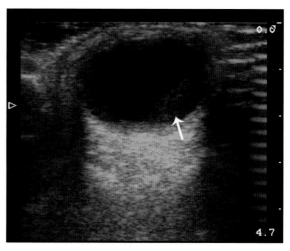

Vitreous hemorrhage: Vitreous hemorrhage (arrow).

Chapter

3

Cardiac ultrasound

Shane Summers

Introduction

Cardiac ultrasound can be used at the bedside in a variety of clinical settings. From the patient with stable vital signs who complains of mild shortness of breath, to the patient with no palpable pulses undergoing CPR. Understanding the mechanics in probe placement is critical to obtaining the necessary view and therefore making an accurate interpretation. Findings on bedside cardiac ultrasound can point the clinician toward a valvular problem, obstructive pathology, or even an infectious etiology.

Normal views

These windows describe the primary locations of transducer placement to visualize the heart through a transthoracic approach.

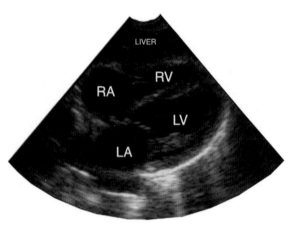

Normal subxiphoid view: In this normal subxiphoid view, all four chambers of the heart are visualized in 1 plane by utilizing the left lobe of the liver as an acoustic window. The subxiphoid approach may be extremely helpful for a global cardiac assessment in a code situation, as it does not interfere with cardiopulmonary resuscitation (CPR). This window may be used to assess for pericardial tamponade, left ventricular (LV) function in shock states, and massive pulmonary embolism with right ventricular (RV) strain. The inferior vena cava may also be interrogated to assess volume status (not depicted).

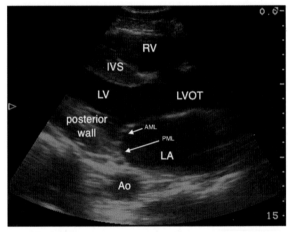

Normal parasternal long-axis (PLAX) view: This normal parasternal long-axis (PLAX) view was obtained by placing the footprint of the transducer at the fourth intercostal space with the indicator pointed to the patient's right shoulder (on cardiac presets). From anterior to posterior, the right ventricle (RV), inter-ventricular septum (IVS), left ventricle (LV), left ventricular outflow tract (LVOT), posterior wall of the LV, anterior and posterior mitral valve leaflets (AML, PML), left atrium (LA), and descending thoracic aorta (Ao) are visualized. The PLAX view can assess for pericardial effusions, LV ejection fraction (LVEF), sequential movement of the mitral and aortic valves, wall motion abnormalities, and dilatation of the aortic root. When the subxiphoid window is unobtainable, the PLAX offers an alternative view for the focused abdominal sonography for trauma (FAST) examination.

Atlas of Emergency Ultrasound, ed. John Christian Fox. Published by Cambridge University Press. © J.C. Fox 2011.

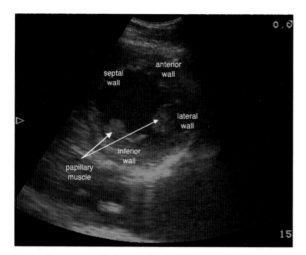

Normal parasternal short-axis view (PSAX) at papillary muscles: The parasternal short-axis view is obtained by placing the transducer just left of the sternum in the third or fourth intercostal space with the indicator pointed to the patient's right shoulder (on cardiac presets). Tilting the transducer toward the apex should reveal a cross-section of the mid left ventricle (LV) and the papillary muscles. This view is useful to observe for assessment of left ventricular ejection fraction (LVEF) as well as wall motion abnormalities in acute myocardial infarctions.

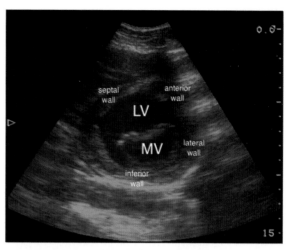

Normal PSAX view at level of the mitral valve: A normal parasternal short-axis window at the mitral valve (MV) level demonstrates a cross-sectional view of the left ventricle (LV) that can be useful for wall motion and ejection fraction assessment. In this plane, the MV has a fish-mouth appearance.

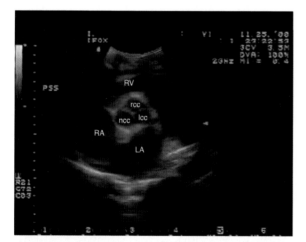

Normal PSAX view at the level of the great vessels: If the transducer is tilted toward the base in a parasternal short-axis view, a cross section of the aortic valve (AV) can be seen. In this patient, a normal tri-leaflet aortic valve is visualized. Note the presence of the non-coronary (NCC), right coronary (RCC), and left coronary cusps (LCC).

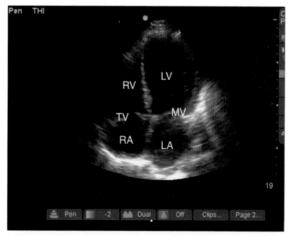

Normal apical four-chamber view (A4C): The apical four-chamber view is obtained by placing the transducer at the point of maximal impulse (PMI) with the indicator pointed to the patient's left lateral chest (on cardiac presets) and the beam directed to the patient's right shoulder. This view is useful for assessment of relative chamber sizes, right (RV) and left ventricular (LV) function, and the atrioventricular valves. This view is optimal for Doppler imaging of the mitral (MV) and tricuspid valves (TV) because blood flow is parallel to the transducer in this plane. This view may also be utilized for an ultrasound guided pericardiocentesis.

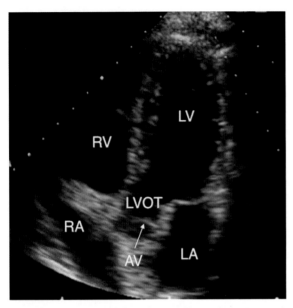

Normal apical five-chamber view (A5C): To obtain the apical five-chamber view, simply tilt the transducer anteriorly from the apical four-chamber view. This view may be helpful to visualize the left ventricular outflow tract and assess function of the aortic valve.

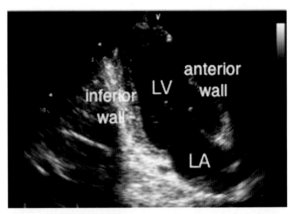

Normal apical two-chamber view (A2C): The apical two-chamber view is obtained by rotating the transducer 75–90 degrees counterclockwise (on cardiac presets) from the apical four-chamber view. This window permits visualization of global left ventricular function and may detect wall motion abnormalities of the anterior and inferior walls.

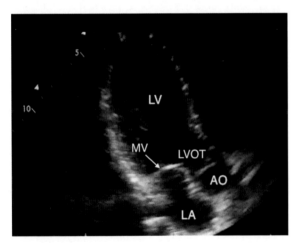

Normal apical long-axis view (A3C): For the apical long (apical three-chamber) view, the indicator is aimed in the same orientation as the parasternal long axis window, but the transducer is instead placed at the apex of the heart (PMI). This view is used to assess global left ventricular (LV) function, the aortic valve, and the left ventricular outflow tract (LVOT).

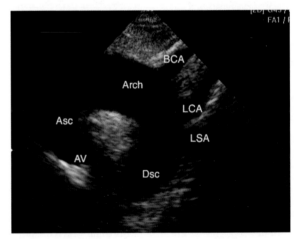

Normal suprasternal view: Although not sensitive, the suprasternal view may be useful to detect proximal aortic dissections. This view is obtained by placing the transducer in the suprasternal notch with the indicator pointing to the patient's left shoulder (on cardiac presets) and the probe angled as anterior as possible. In this plane, the aortic valve (AV), ascending aorta (Asc), aortic arch (Arch), descending thoracic aorta (Dsc), brachiocephalic (BCA) artery, left common carotid artery (LCA), and left subclavian artery (LSA) are seen.

Pericardial effusion versus pericardial tamponade

This set of images describe the findings seen to differentiate simple fluid collections around the heart to obstructive tamponade.

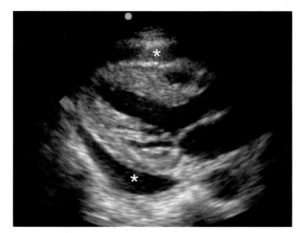

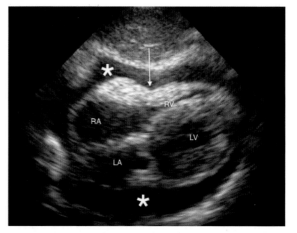

Large circumferential pericardial effusion: Parasternal long axis view is remarkable for a circumferential pericardial effusion (asterisks) in a patient with malignancy. Note that there is greater than 1 cm of echolucent space between the visceral and parietal pericardium both anterior and posterior (asterisks) consistent with a large effusion.

Cardiac tamponade with diastolic right ventricle collapse: Subxiphoid view in a patient with systemic lupus erythematosus (SLE) reveals a circumferential pericardial effusion (asterisks) with collapse of the right ventricular free wall during diastole (arrow) and near obliteration of the RV lumen, consistent with pericardial tamponade.

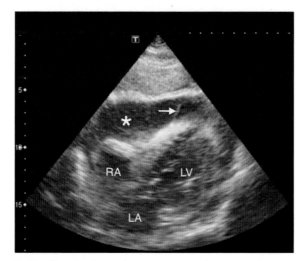

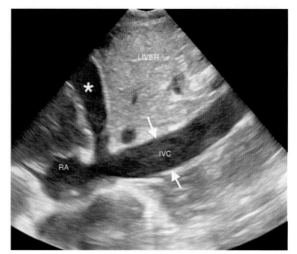

Pericardiocentesis: In the same patient with an SLE and pericardial tamponade, a pericardiocentesis is attempted using a subxiphoid approach. The hyperechoic reverberating needle (arrow) can be seen entering the pericardial space (asterisk) under ultrasound guidance.

Cardiac tamponade with plethoric inferior vena cava: In a patient with a large pericardial effusion (asterisk), a subxiphoid view of the inferior vena cava (IVC) is remarkable for a plethoric IVC (arrows) greater than 2.5 cm in diameter with no collapse at end inspiration, consistent with a central venous pressure greater than 20 mm Hg and pericardial tamponade.

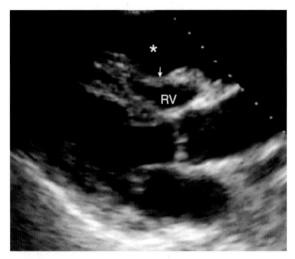

Cardiac tamponade with anterior pericardial effusion: In a long-axis view obtained for a patient with undifferentiated hypotension, and anterior pericardial effusion (asterisk) is collapsing the free wall of the right ventricle during diastole (arrow), nearly obliterating the RV lumen and leading to pericardial tamponade.

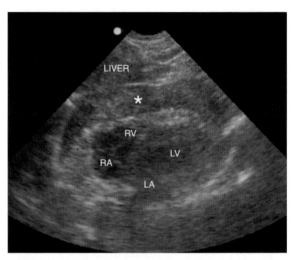

Hemopericardium: This subxiphoid image was obtained in a patient with a transmediastinal gunshot wound and cardiac arrest. Echogenic material was noted in the pericardial space with severely depressed cardiac contractility. An immediate bedside thoracotomy was performed with evacuation of pericardial clot.

Enlargement

These images demonstrate the pathology encountered when hypertrophy and dilation are encountered.

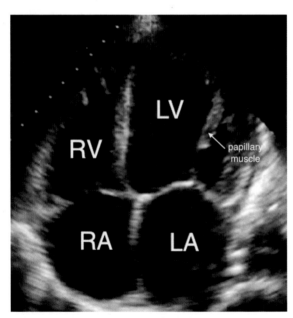

Dilated cardiomyopathy: Apical four-chamber view in an alcoholic patient with decompensated heart failure is remarkable for a dilated cardiomyopathy. Note the globular shape to the left ventricle (LV), thin walls, and biatrial enlargement. Real-time echocardiography revealed little change in LV diameter from diastole to systole consistent with severely depressed ejection fraction (EF).

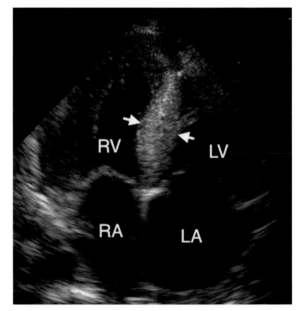

Hypertrophic obstructive cardiomyopathy (HOCM): An apical four-chamber view of the heart is obtained in the emergency department for a patient with exertional syncope and a heart murmur. The bedside exam was remarkable for a significantly thickened interventricular septum consistent with hypertrophic cardiomyopathy.

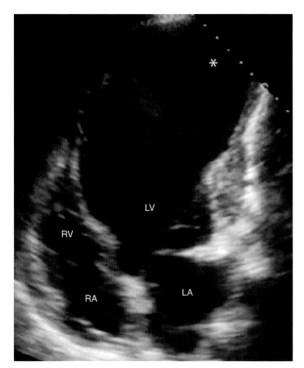

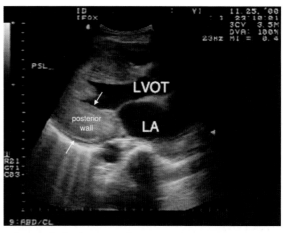

Left ventricular hypertrophy: Parasternal long-axis view of the heart in a patient with poorly controlled hypertension reveals left ventricular (LV) hypertrophy. In end diastole, the wall thickness of the posterior wall of the LV (arrows) measured greater than 3 cm.

Apical left ventricular aneurysm: An apical four-chamber view of the heart is remarkable for a large apical aneurysm (*). The patient was status post acute myocardial infarction with pathologic Q waves and ST segment elevation on EKG.

Right heart strain

This may be the only clue to diagnosing a pulmonary embolism in the setting of cardiovascular collapse. Thrombolitics are indicated for pulmonary embolism in the setting of shock.

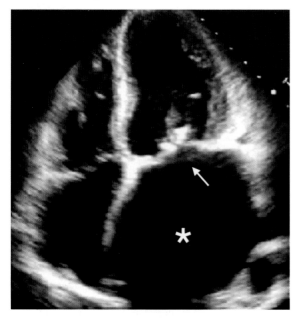

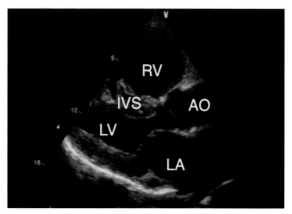

Massive pulmonary embolism with acute right heart strain: In this parasternal long-axis view of a patient with massive pulmonary embolism (PE), a dilated right ventricle (RV) is apparent consistent with right heart strain. Generally, a normal ratio of chamber sizes measured across the tips of atrioventricular (AV) valves is RV:LV 0.6:1. Although no finding is sufficiently sensitive to exclude PE, other echocardiographic findings include direct visualization of the clot, paradoxical motion of the interventricular septum (IVS) from elevated right heart pressures, and tricuspid regurgitation.

Mitral stenosis with left atrial enlargement: In a patient with rheumatic heart disease and severe mitral stenosis (arrow), a grossly enlarged left atrium is visualized on an apical four-chamber view (asterisk).

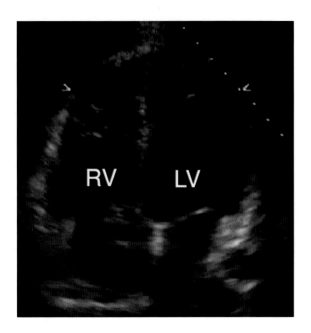

Massive pulmonary embolism in pulseless electrical activity (PEA) arrest: An apical four-chamber view of the heart obtained in a patient with pulseless electrical activity (PEA) arrest and massive pulmonary embolism. Note the right ventricular (RV) diameter approaches that of the left ventricle, and the RV free wall is rounded in shape. On real-time echocardiography, a severely dyskinetic RV was apparent, and RV function improved after intravenous administration of tissue plasminogen activator (tPA).

Valvular dysfunction

Using colorflow, one can appreciate the presence and severity of valvular pathology.

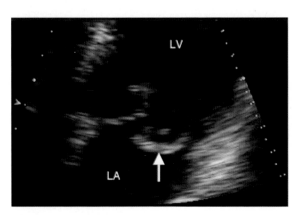

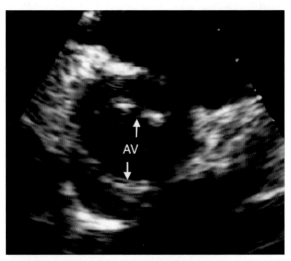

Mitral valve prolapse: In this apical four-chamber view with zoom on the left heart, abnormal motion of the posterior leaflet of the mitral valve (arrow) with prolapse into the left atrium (LA) is apparent.

Bicuspid aortic valve: In a zoomed parasternal short-axis view at the base obtained in a patient with chest pain and syncope, a bicuspid aortic valve is visualized (arrows).

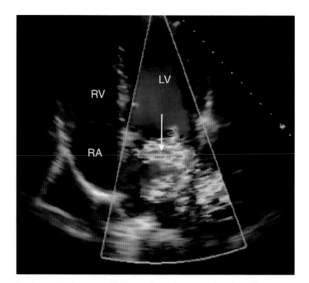

Acute mitral regurgitation: An apical four-chamber view is obtained in a patient with decompensated heart failure from ruptured papillary muscle. Color Doppler placed across the mitral valve reveals severe mitral regurgitation with retrograde turbulent flow during systole. In variance mode, turbulent (non-laminar) flow demonstrates a mosaic pattern of turquoise and yellow pixels (arrow).

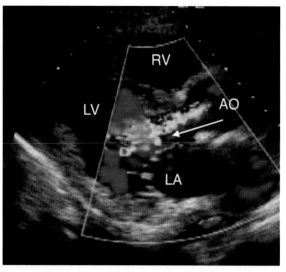

Acute aortic regurgitation: A parasternal long-axis view is remarkable for turbulent flow (mosaic appearance) across the aortic valve (arrow) during diastole in a patient with severe aortic regurgitation.

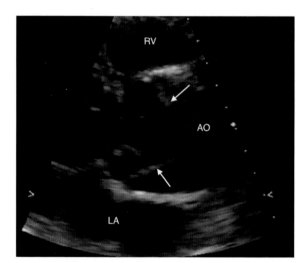

Proximal aortic dissection: Parasternal long-axis view of the heart demonstrates an intimal flap (arrows) and dilated aortic root consistent with proximal aortic dissection. Although transthoracic echocardiography (TEE) is not sufficiently sensitive to exclude aortic dissection, early diagnosis on bedside ultrasound can facilitate mobilization of resources and expedite treatment.

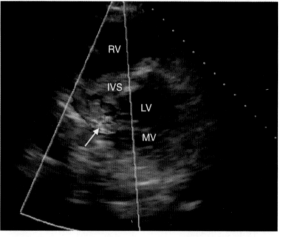

Ventricular septal defect: A parasternal short-axis view at the mitral valve (MV) level reveals turbulent flow with mosaic color Doppler signal (arrow) across the interventricular septum (IVS) consistent with a ventricular septal defect.

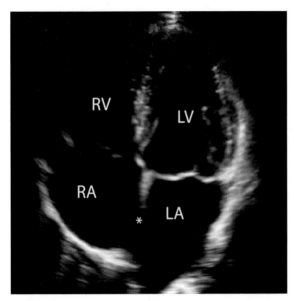

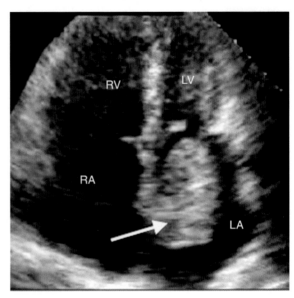

Atrial septal defect: On B mode imaging, apical four-chamber view of the heart reveals an atrial septal defect (ASD, asterisk). Note right atrial enlargement from left-to-right shunting. Other clues for the presence of an ASD may include right ventricular hypertrophy and paradoxical motion of the ventricular septum. Color flow Doppler can confirm the diagnosis, determine flow direction, and estimate the size of the defect.

Atrial myxoma: On an apical four-chamber view, a large echogenic mass is visualized in the left atrium consistent with atrial myxoma (arrow).

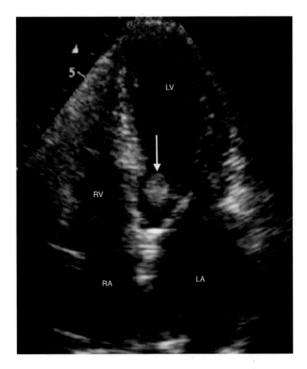

Acute infective endocarditis: In an intravenous drug abuser with fever of unknown origin, an apical four-chamber view reveals a discrete pedunculated vegetation on the anterior leaflet of the mitral valve consistent with infective endocarditis.

Ultrasound of the lung

Justin Davis and Seric Cusick

Normal lung

Sonographic interrogation of the thoracic cavity involves interpretation of anatomic structures as well as the recognition of the presence/absence of several artifacts. This may be facilitated by the use of M-mode and color Doppler. A variety of transducers may be employed, including phased, convex, and linear. The resolution of linear transducers is preferred by some for characterization of pleural movement and artifacts arising at this level. However, phased and convex array transducers with a lower frequency offer greater penetration, allowing identification of deeper pathology and appreciation of further artifacts.

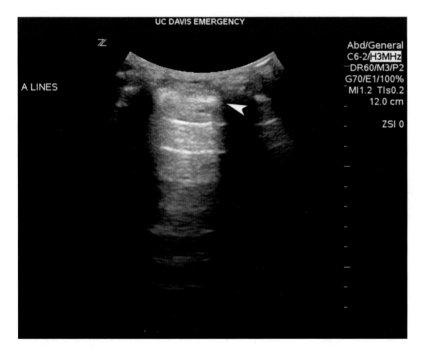

Normal lung, curvilinear: Normal lung imaged with curvilinear probe. Again note the ribs with acoustic shadows, the pleural line (arrowhead) and multiple horizontal A-lines.

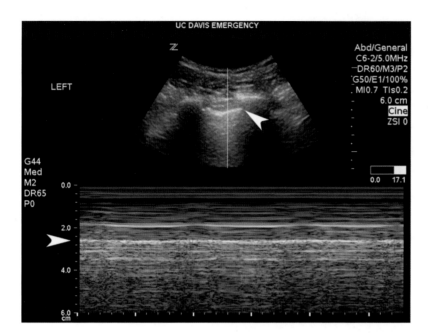

Normal lung, curvilinear, M-mode: Normal lung, curvilinear probe in M-mode (time-motion mode) showing the "seashore sign" of normal lung sliding. Above the pleural line (arrowheads) the image is constant while below it is constantly changing, reflecting the shifting artifacts seen as pleura slide past one another.

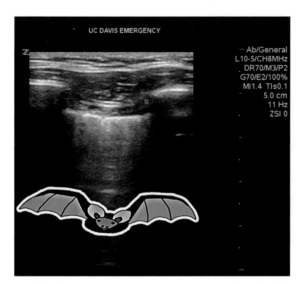

Normal lung, linear: Normal lung ultrasound anatomy. Two ribs in cross-section are used as landmarks to find the pleura; as the pleura must run in a line connecting their interior surface. The hyperechoic ribs and pleural line together form a shape suggestive of a bat flying toward the viewer; with the body as the pleura and wings as the ribs (the "bat sign").

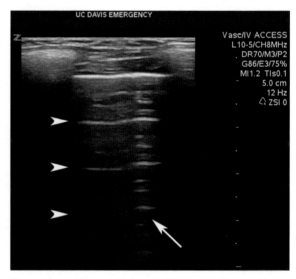

Normal lung, linear, A-line and Z-line: Normal lung with multiple horizontal A-line artifacts (arrowheads). Running vertically is a Z-line, which arises from the pleura, enhances the A-lines and does not extend to the edge of the screen.

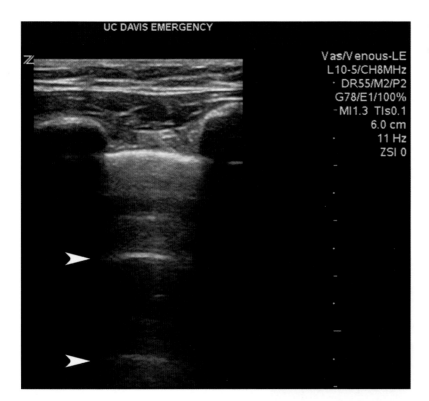

Normal lung, linear, A-line: Normal lung with a linear probe. A-lines are again seen (arrowheads).

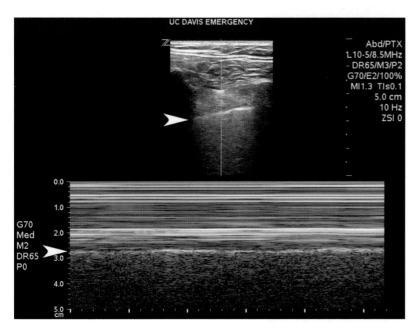

Normal lung, linear, M-mode: Normal lung, linear probe in M-mode. The seashore sign representing normal lung sliding, with the changing artifacts below the pleural line (arrowheads).

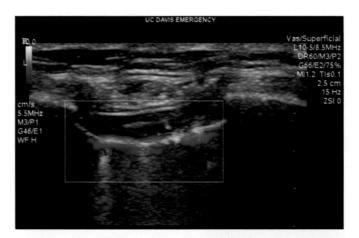

Normal lung, linear, color power Doppler: Normal lung, color power Doppler. Another way to view lung sliding is to place power Doppler over the pleural line. The movement causes localized Doppler artifacts along the pleural line, known as the "power slide" sign.

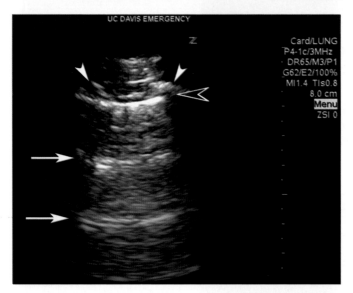

Normal lung, phased array, A-lines: Normal lung. Note the ribs (arrowheads) with the acoustic shadows deep to them. Reflected sound reverberates between the pleural line (clear arrowhead) and the transducer, creating multiple horizontal artifacts called A-lines (arrows).

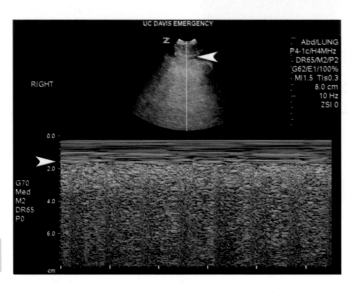

Normal lung, phased array, M-mode: Normal lung imaged with phased array probe in M-mode. Again, the seashore sign is seen with the motion artifacts deep to the pleural line (arrowheads).

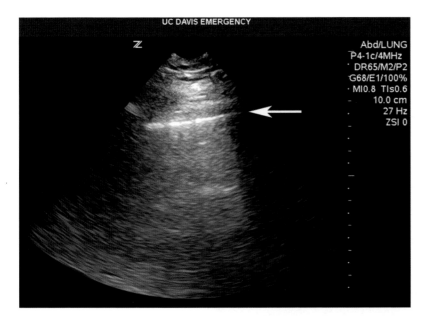

Normal lung, phased array, O-lines: Normal lung imaged with phased array probe. Below the pleural line (arrow) there are no significant A-lines seen; but rather a gray haze; sometimes referred to as a collection of O-lines. Slight movement of the probe will often demonstrate A-lines.

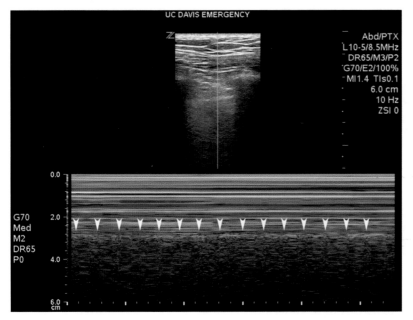

Normal lung, M-mode, lung pulse: Non-ventilated lung, M-mode. When the lung is not expanding with respiration, the M-mode shows the sign known as the "lung pulse," with rhythmic artifacts below the pleural line that correspond to translated motion from the heart. This is seen in the non-ventilated lung after main-stem intubation, severe atelectasis, or apnea as demonstrated here with both a linear and phased array transducer.

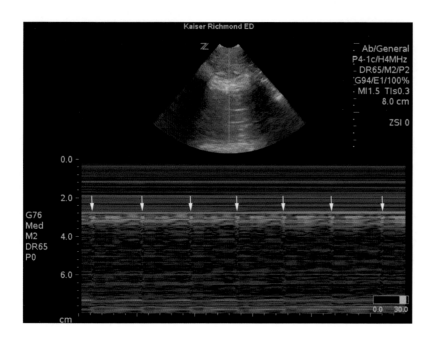

Normal lung, M-mode, lung pulse: (*cont.*)

Pneumothorax

Identification of a pneumothorax with ultrasound relies upon the absence of normal lung sliding and comet-tail artifacts. Findings on M-mode and color power Doppler may assist in identifying this. While the absence of these features is sensitive for pneumothorax, only the identification of a lung point provides good specificity.

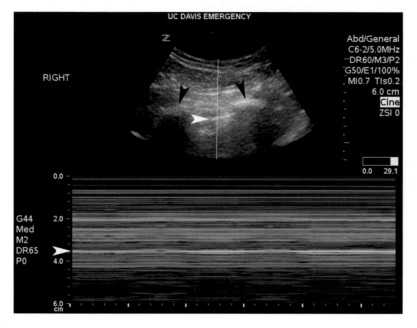

Pneumothorax, curvilinear, M-mode: Pneumothorax, M-mode. The ribs (black arrowheads) frame the pleura (white arrowhead). Rather than the normal "seashore sign" here we see the "stratosphere sign."

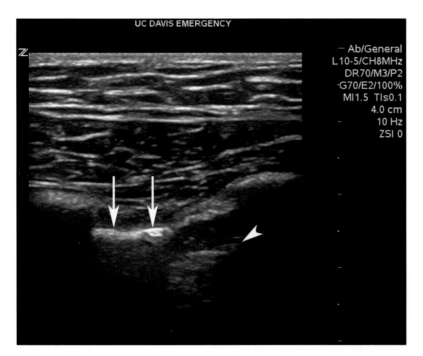

Normal lung, linear, false lung point: Normal lung edge. A common reason for a false-positive pneumothorax finding is the misinterpretation of a lung edge adjacent to the diaphragm, pericardium, or effusion as a "lung point." Here, the pleural line of the normal lung edge (arrows) is seen to dynamically obscure the pericardium (arrowhead). In a pneumothorax, the area adjacent to the "lung point" must be a continuation of a bright pleural line, usually with A-lines below it. In this example, the bright pleural line of the aerated lung edge does not continue, showing that the mobile lung is not displacing air as it slides along the chest wall, but rather tissue or fluid.

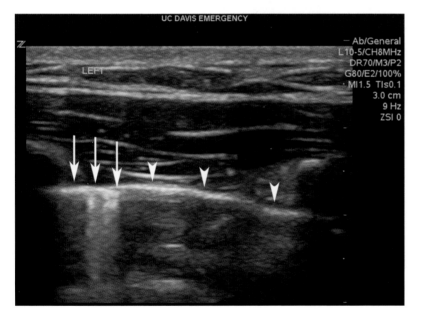

Pneumothorax, linear, lung point: The right side of the image shows the pleural line (arrowheads) that is lacking normal lung sliding on real-time imaging. The left side shows intermittent lung sliding (arrows) that appears and disappears. Known as a "lung point," this represents an area of lung that intermittently touches the parietal pleura and is considered 100% specific for pneumothorax.

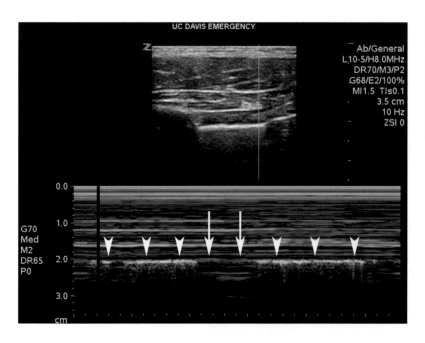

Normal lung, linear, M-mode, false lung point: Note the intermittent "seashore sign" of sliding aerated lung (arrowheads). In contrast to the "lung point" of pneumothorax, here in the intervening period the bright white pleural line disappears entirely (arrows) and the deeper pericardium is visible. Increasing the depth would make the lung pericardial motion more apparent.

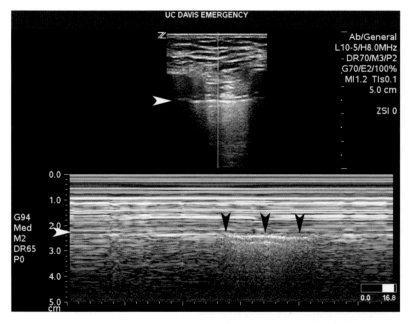

Pneumothorax, linear, M-mode, lung point: The "stratosphere sign" is again seen below the pleural line (white arrowheads), but this time is momentarily interrupted by a return of the "seashore sign" (black arrowheads) as the collapsed lung touches the chest wall with inspiration. This transition is known as a "lung point" and is considered 100% specific for pneumothorax.

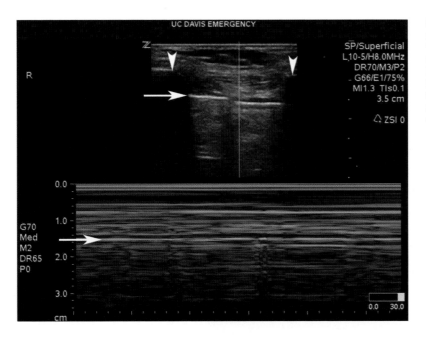

Pneumothorax, linear, M-mode: The normal "seashore sign" is replaced by the "stratosphere sign" or "barcode sign" in this image. The ribs (arrowheads) are landmarks for locating the parietal pleura (arrow). Below the pleural line, note the absence of the normal motion artifacts, resembling either many planes leaving contrails in the sky or a retail barcode.

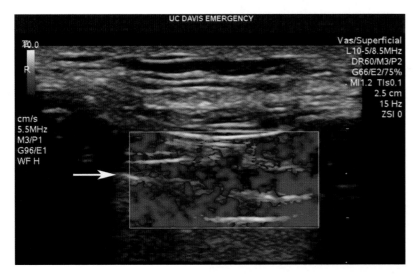

Pneumothorax, linear, color power Doppler: Power Doppler imaging shows a lack of expected motion artifact along the pleural line (arrow), but rather a diffuse flash artifact as the Doppler gain is increased.

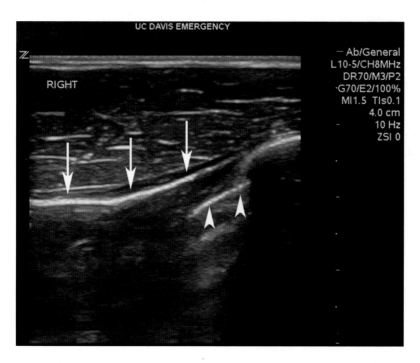

Subcutaneous air, linear: A common pitfall of beginning sonographers is to mistake subcutaneous air for a pneumothorax. Like a pneumothorax, air in the chest wall has no lung sliding and will show a "stratosphere sign" on M-mode. The key to recognition is to always start with identification of the ribs. The pleural line (arrowheads) resides at the level of the deep rib surface, while subcutaneous air (arrows) will be superficial to this.

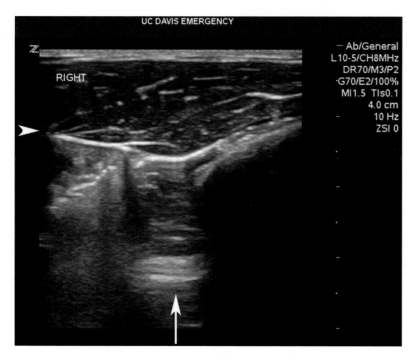

Subcutaneous air, linear, E-line: The bright line of subcutaneous air (arrowhead) is distinguished from the pleural line by noting that it is even with the superficial surface of the rib shown at right. An E-line (arrow) is seen echoing downward and has similar appearance to a B-line, except that it arises from emphysema rather than from a pleural line.

Interstitial syndrome

Fluid in the interlobular septae extends to the visceral pleura, creating a pathway for sound waves to enter and become reflected repeatedly between adjacent alveoli like a hall of mirrors. The escaping echoes create hyperechoic artifacts known as B-lines. B-lines arise from the pleura, extend to the edge of the image, erase normal A-lines, and move with lung sliding.

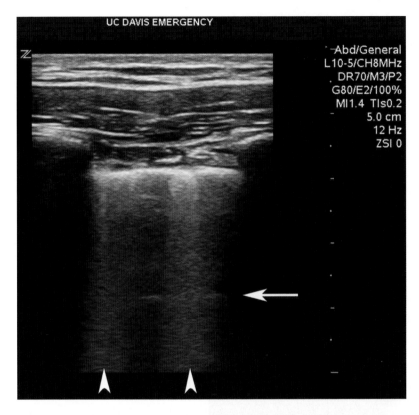

Interstitial syndrome, linear: B-Lines (arrowheads) arise from the pleura; obliterate A-lines (arrow); extend to the edge of the image; and move with lung sliding. Rare isolated B-lines can be seen in normal lungs.

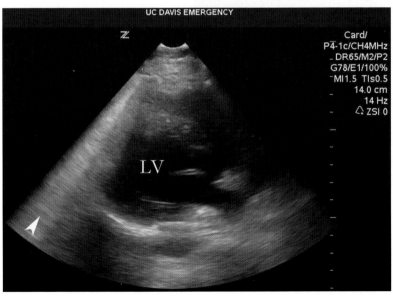

Interstitial syndrome, phased array: At times, information on the lungs can be obtained while performing other studies, as in this parasternal long axis cardiac window. In these two images, multiple B-lines (arrowheads) move with respiration to obscure varying amounts of the left ventricle (LV).

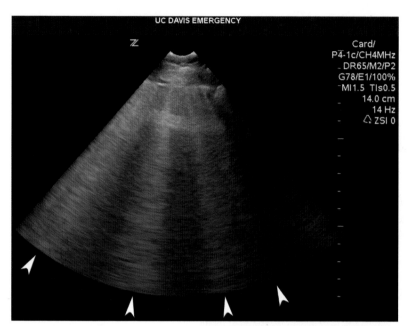

Interstitial syndrome, phased array: (cont.)

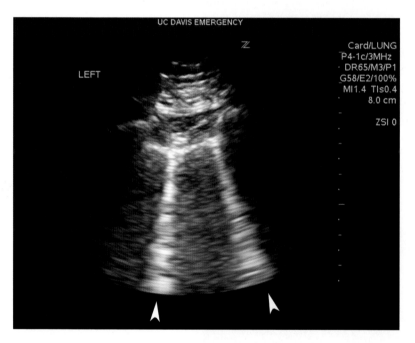

Interstitial syndrome, phased array: Note the absence of A-lines.

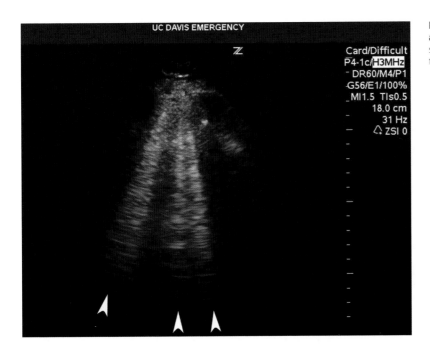

Interstitial syndrome, phased array: Three B-lines (arrowheads) are seen extending from the pleural line to the periphery.

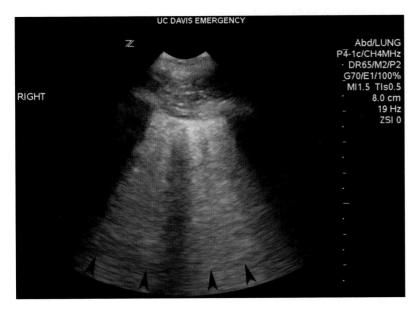

Alveolar interstitial syndrome, phased array: Multiple B-lines (arrowheads) are seen to converge into a nearly "white lung."

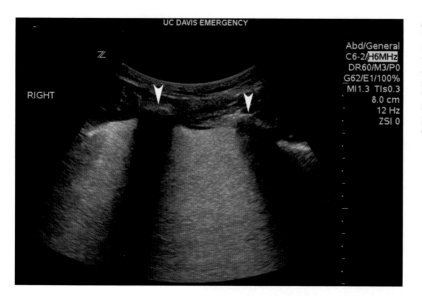

Alveolar interstitial syndrome: The two ribs (arrowheads) cast dense shadows, while the lung shows a diffuse white artifact, consistent with a confluence of B-lines. This "white lung" is seen in conditions that cause a peripheral "ground glass" infiltrate on CT scan, including lung contusion (this image), pneumonia, infarction, diffuse interstitial disease, and ARDS.

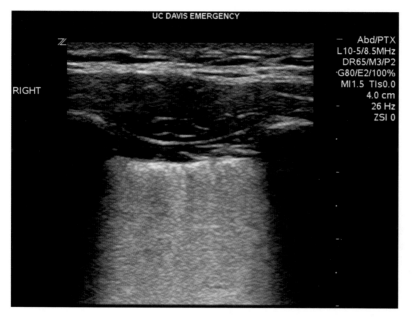

Alveolar interstitial syndrome, linear: Another example of the "white lung" sign seen in a blunt trauma patient with a focal lung contusion.

Alveolar consolidation

Consolidations may be identified with ultrasound as segments of lung adjacent to the parietal pleura develop an increasing proportion of fluid and pulmonary parenchyma relative to air.

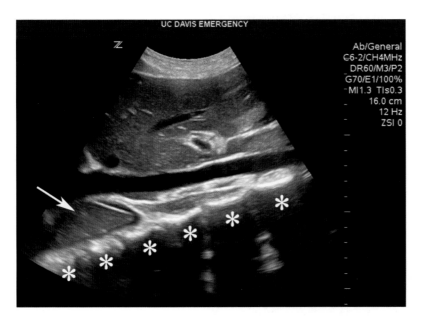

Alveolar consolidation of the right lung base: The right lung (arrow) shows "hepatization" in this longitudinal view of the inferior vena cava. The spine shadows (asterisks) continue above the diaphragm and are clearly visualized into the thorax. This "spine sign" requires the absence of normal air-induced mirror image artifacts across the diaphragm and indicates either effusion, consolidation, or both.

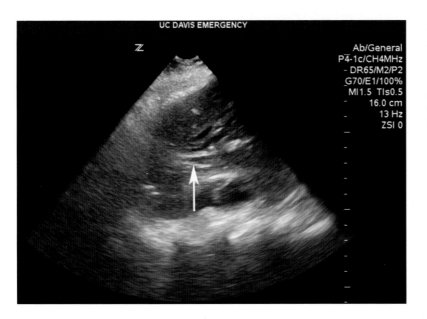

Alveolar consolidation with dynamic air bronchogram: In these two images, the lung base shows minimal aeration. When observed in real-time, air (arrowheads) is seen to move back and forth through the bronchial tree (arrow) with respiratory effort, very suggestive of pneumonia over atelectasis.

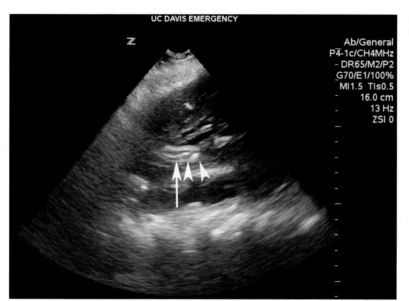

Alveolar consolidation with dynamic air bronchogram: *(cont.)*

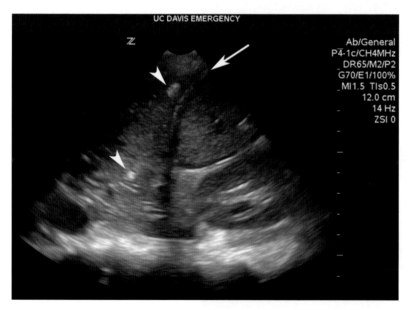

Alveolar consolidation of the left lung base, left coronal view: The diaphragm (arrow) overlying the spleen provides the landmark for viewing the lung base. The lung is consolidated and nearly void of air, with the exception of two air bronchograms (arrowheads). There is also a small effusion and a positive "spine sign."

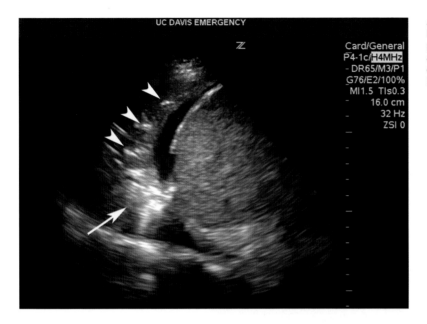

Alveolar consolidation of the right lung base with effusion: Several pinpoint air bronchograms (arrowheads) are seen amid the "hepatized" lung. The deep portion exhibits the ragged aerated border of the "shred sign" (arrow).

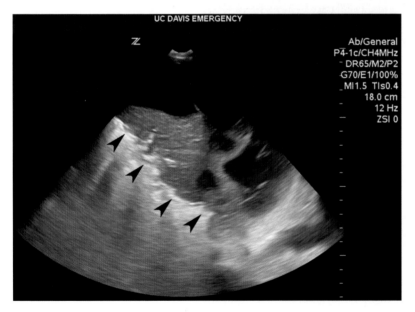

Alveolar consolidation with effusion: The aerated lung forms an irregular deep border (arrowheads) to the consolidated gray lung tissue, known as the "shred sign" due to the border's irregular appearance.

Pleural effusion

Identification of pleural effusions with ultrasound has implications for both diagnosis and procedural guidance. Coronal views (as used in the Focused Assessment with Sonography in Trauma) provide interrogation of the dependent portions of the thoracic cavity in the supine patient.

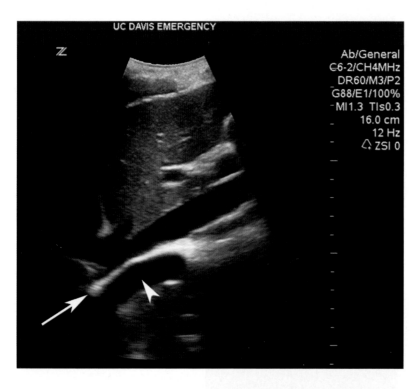

Normal lung with mirror-image artifact, longitudinal subxiphoid view: The smooth and bright pleural line (arrow) creates a mirror artifact (arrowhead) of the IVC, potentially leading to a false-positive finding of right pleural effusion.

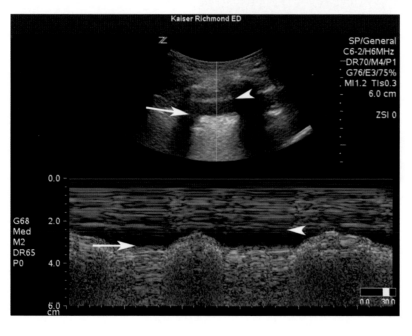

Pleural effusion, M-mode: A hypoechoic fluid collection separates the lung surface (arrows) and the parietal pleura (arrowheads). The lung rises and falls with respiration; creating the "sinusoid sign."

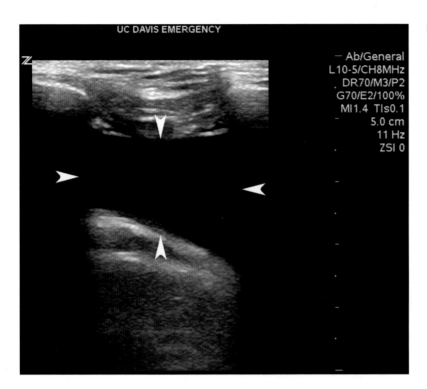

Pleural effusion: The effusion appears to be bordered on four sides (arrowheads) by the lung, chest wall, and rib shadows, referred to as the "quad sign."

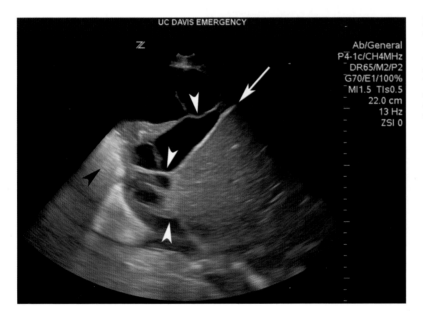

Pleural effusion with fibrinous debris, right coronal view: The hypoechoic collection over the diaphragm (arrow) contains cordlike debris (white arrowheads) that appears to tether the consolidated lung (black arrowhead) to the parietal pleura. Such debris and adhesions are less reliably visualized by CT.

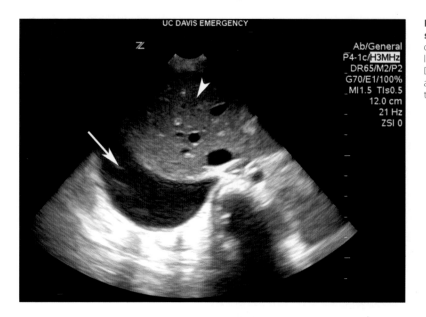

Right pleural effusion, transverse subxiphoid view: A hypoechoic collection (arrow) is seen deep to the liver (arrowhead) at the right thorax base. Due to interference from bowel gas and image depth, this view is less reliable than lateral coronal or posterior views.

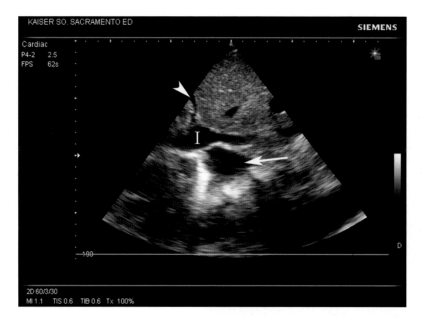

Right pleural effusion and small pericardial effusion, subxiphoid longitudinal view: The IVC (I) runs through the diaphragm separating the right basilar plural effusion (arrow) and small pericardial effusion (arrowhead).

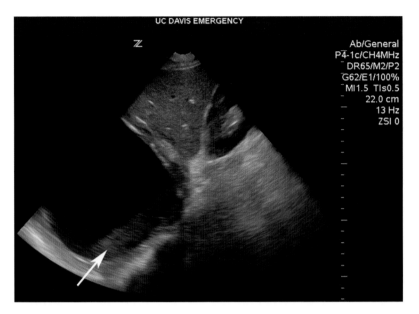

Large right loculated empyema: Above the diaphragm, a well-contained hypoechoic fluid collection has layering debris (arrow). Color Doppler of the encircling tissue can help differentiate empyema from intraparenchymal abscess (not shown).

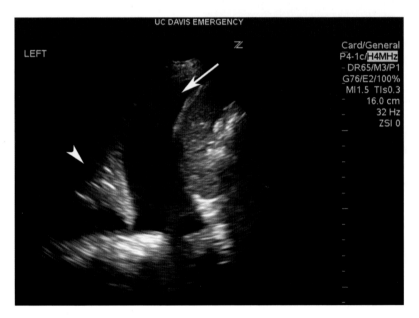

Left pleural effusion, coronal view: A large effusion (arrow) is seen above the diaphragm, with a consolidated lower lobe edge (arrowhead) floating in the fluid, moving with inspiration on real-time imaging.

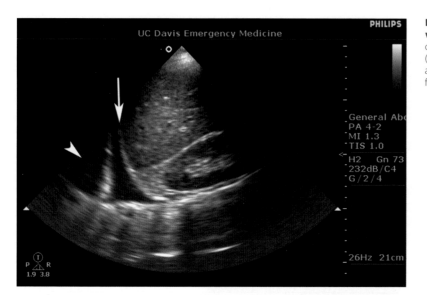

Left basilar pleural effusion, coronal view: A small hypoechoic fluid collection is seen above the diaphragm (arrow). Under real-time imaging, the aerated lung (arrowhead) is seen to follow diaphragmatic excursion.

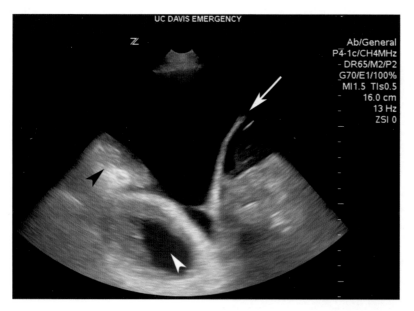

Left pleural effusion, posterior sagittal view: A large effusion is seen over the diaphragm (arrow), pushing aside the consolidated lung (black arrowhead) in preparation for thoracentesis. Thoracentesis at this rib space would endanger neither the diaphragm nor the lung. With large effusions, the heart (white arrowhead) can sometimes be seen from posterior windows.

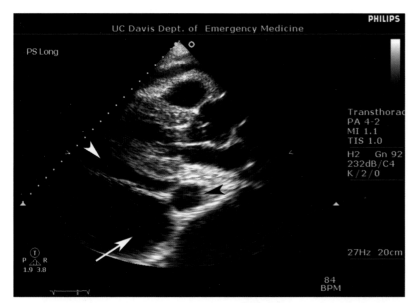

Left pleural effusion and pericardial effusion, parasternal long-axis cardiac view: A pericardial effusion (arrowhead) lies anterior to the descending aorta (black arrowhead) while a large left pleural effusion (arrow) is found posterior to the aorta.

Right upper quadrant ultrasonography
Post injury intervals

Daniel Gromis and John Christian Fox

Anatomy

Biliary anatomy is important to identify and can be difficult to orient to. The utilization of landmarks and color flow or power Doppler are effective tools in delineating structures and localizing structures accurately.

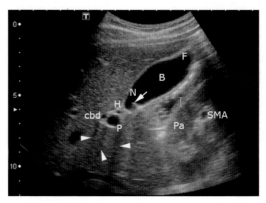

Anatomy, Mickey Mouse sign: The "Mickey Mouse sign" is composed of the hepatic artery (H), portal vein (P), and common bile duct (cbd). The neck (N) and body (B) of the gallbladder are divided by the neck fold (arrow), with the fundus (F) lying most anteriorly. The shadowing cast (arrowheads) is as a result of edge refraction. Pancreas (Pa), superior mesenteric artery (SMA).

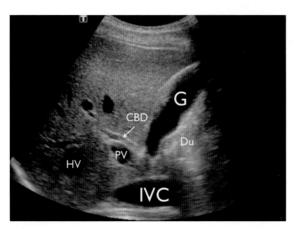

Anatomy: The gallbladder (G) is the most anterior structure, lateral to the duodenum (Du) on sagittal imaging, and overlying the common bile duct (CBD), and portal vein (PV). More laterally, also seen is the short axis of the hepatic vein (HV). In the far field at the bottom of the image is the inferior vena cava (IVC).

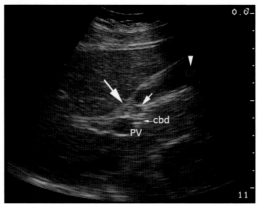

Anatomy, main lobar fissure: Identification of the main lobar fissure (large arrow) orients to the gallbladder with its fundal stone (arrowhead), common bile duct (cbd), and portal vein (PV). Neck fold (small arrow).

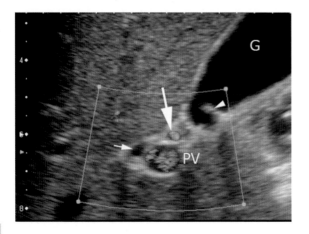

Anatomy, Mickey Mouse sign: Color Doppler, short axis imaging of the Mickey Mouse sign showing a strong signal in the hepatic artery (large arrow) and portal vein (PV), but a lack of flow in the common bile duct (small arrow). Gallbladder (G), neck fold (arrowhead).

Atlas of Emergency Ultrasound, ed. John Christian Fox. Published by Cambridge University Press. © J.C. Fox 2011.

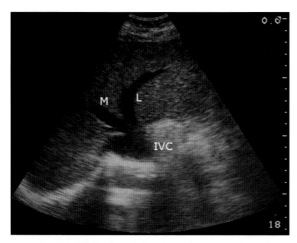

Anatomy, vascular: The "Playboy Bunny sign" is made up of the inferior vena cava (IVC) and middle (M) and left (L) hepatic veins when the liver is viewed obliquely.

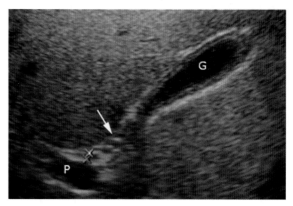

Anatomy, cystic duct: The cystic duct (arrow) with its spiral valves seen connecting the gallbladder (G) to common bile duct (bordered by x's) commonly casts a shadow artifact. Portal vein (P). This gallbladder is contracted.

Cholelithiasis

Gallstones are the most common pathology to the gallbladder. Their location, size, quantity, and characteristics should be noted, as each conveys different significance to the diagnostic workup.

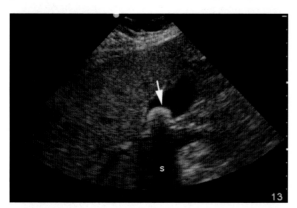

Cholelithiasis: A large gallstone (arrow) with classic anterior hyperechogenicity and clean distal acoustic shadowing (s).

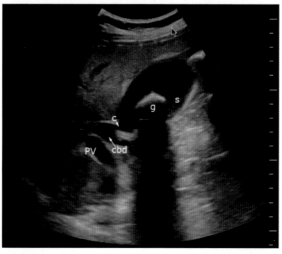

Large stone: A large stone (g) dependently oriented superior to biliary sludge (s). Cysti duct (c), common bile duct (cbd), portal vein (PV).

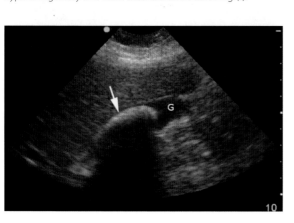

Large stone: A massive stone (arrow) casts its hypoechogenic shadow as a result of sound wave reflection, while the fluid-filled gallbladder lumen (G) causes far-field attenuation and hyperechogenicity.

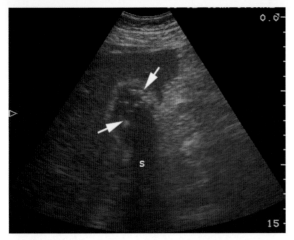

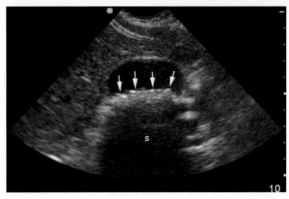

Multiple stones: The arrows indicate multiple stones dispersed within the gallbladder lumen with subsequent cumulative distal acoustic shadowing (s).

Multiple stones: The arrows identify a multitude of stones laying along the floor of the gallbladder with a resultant aggregate distal acoustic shadowing (s).

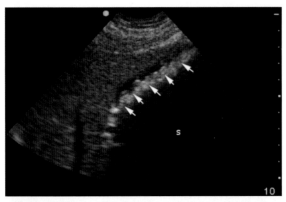

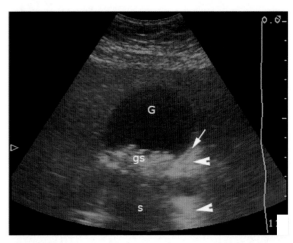

Multiple stones: Arrows show layering of multiple tiny stones with near obliteration of the gallbladder lumen, seen as a sliver of hypoechogenicity anteriorly overlying the hyperechoic stones. The farfield aggregate shadow (s) cast by the stones can be seen.

Multiple stones: Seen in a sagittal dimension, the gallbladder (G) has multiple stones (gs) posteriorly casting a far-field shadow (s). Acoustic enhancement (arrowheads) from the fluid-filled gallbladder illuminates the pericholecystic fluid (arrow).

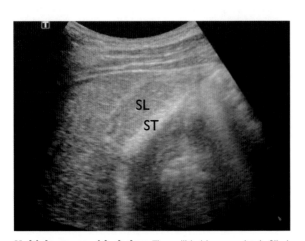

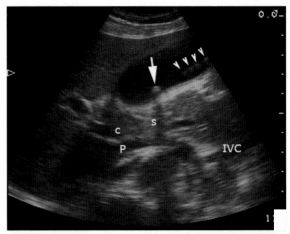

Multiple stones with sludge: The gallbladder, completely filled with isoechoic sludge (SL) is seen anterior to multiple aggregated gallstones (GS) collecting along the posterior gallbladder.

Gallstone locations: The four, non-shadowing stones near the gallbladder fundus (arrowheads) demonstrate the "peas in a pod" formation. The single large stone (arrow) is more heavily calcified and casts a clean shadow (s). Common bile duct (c), portal vein (P), inferior vena cava (IVC).

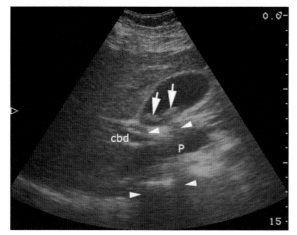

Gallstone locations: Two large stones (arrows), confirmed by their respective far-field shadowing (arrowheads) can be seen in the neck of the gallbladder. Common bile duct (cbd), portal vein (P).

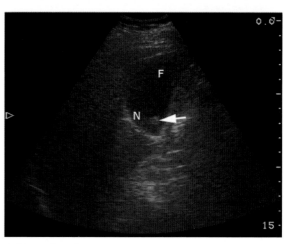

Gallstone locations: A hyperechoic stone (arrow) located in the gallbladder neck (N), posterior to the fundus (F) in sagittal section.

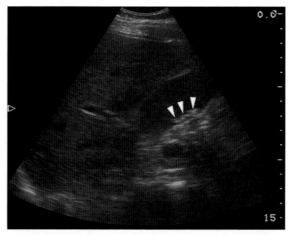

Gallstone locations: A collection of "peas in a pod" gallstones (arrowheads) without distal shadowing seen in the body of the gallbladder.

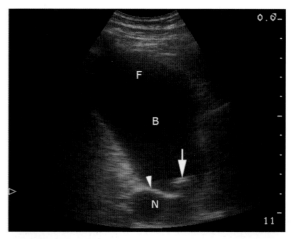

Missed stones: A non-shadowing stone (arrow) is noted atop the neck fold (arrowhead) of the gallbladder. Fundus (F), body (B), neck (N).

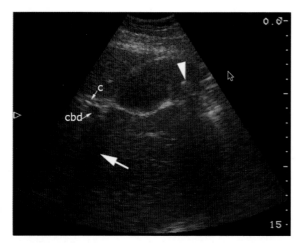

Missed stones, edge refraction shadowing: A gallstone (arrowhead) could easily be missed if not carefully scrutinized for its anterior hyperechogenicity seen at the tip of the arrowhead. A shadow (arrow) falsely identifies a stone at the gallbladder neck, and instead represents edge refraction shadowing caused by the cystic duct (c). Common bile duct (cbd).

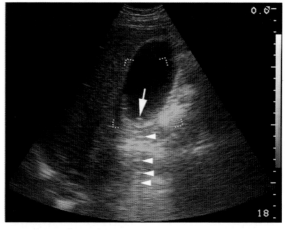

Missed stones, reverberation artifact: Heavily calcified stones (arrow) occasionally fail to produce an acoustic shadow, but rather display hyperechoic, acoustic reverberation (arrowheads). The degree of pronouncement of the reverberations is thought to be proportional to the degree of calcification of the stone.

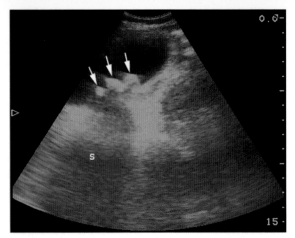

Missed stones, over-gaining: When over-gained, gallstones (arrows) only produce faint shadowing (s), which could easily be missed and elucidates the importance of appropriate gain calibration.

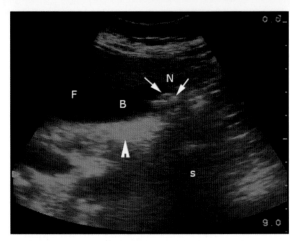

Missed stones, neck clustering: When multiple stones (arrows) aggregate in the gallbladder neck (N), the resultant shadow (s) can be misinterpreted as edge refraction shadowing if the gallbladder is not carefully scrutinized. Fundus (F), body (B), acoustic enhancement (arrowhead).

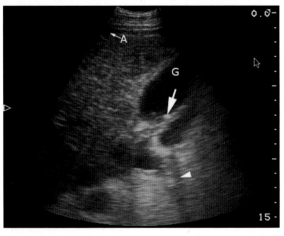

Missed stones, lost shadow: A small, single stone (arrow) casts a very small shadow (arrowhead), which can be easily missed, especially when cast through equally hypoechogenic structures. Ascites (A).

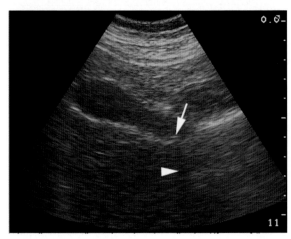

Missed stones, tiny stone: A very small stone (arrow) casts a fine shadow (arrowhead) from the gallbladder neck (N).

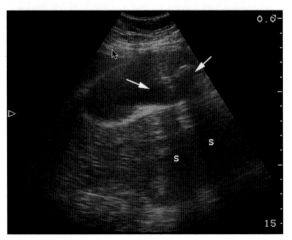

Missed stones, shadows: Occasionally, even large stones (arrows) are difficult to identify, save for their far-field shadows (s).

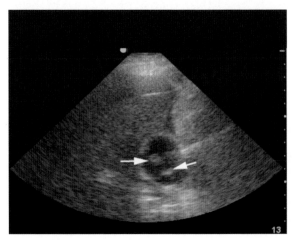

Missed stones, floating stones: When the specific gravity of bile is increased – by ingestion of contrast media or extensive biliary sludging, stones (arrows) can float in the medium and be missed.

Common bile duct

The common bile duct (CBD) is one of the most important, although often most difficult, structures to identify when imaging the right upper quadrant on a patient in whom a provider has concern for biliary pathology. Care should be taken to identify the portal vein, atop which lies the common bile duct.

Once identified, the internal luminal diameter should be carefully measured. A patient can be considered to have a normally sized common bile duct if this diameter is approximately 1 mm for every decade of life, but generally considered dilated once it exceeds 6 mm.

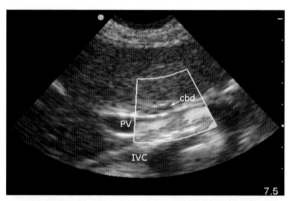

Normal CBD: Power Doppler sonography demonstrates flow in the portal vein and a lack of flow in the anteriorly overlying common bile duct.

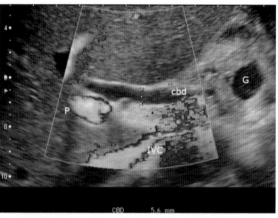

CBD thickening: Under power Doppler sonography, the internal diameter of the common bile duct (cbd) lumen is seen to measure 5.6 mm. Gallbladder (G), portal vein (P), inferior vena cava (IVC).

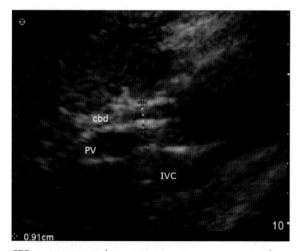

CBD measurement, inaccurate: Improper measurement of the cbd. The calipers (x's) are seen measuring the diameter of the walls to 0.91 cm, but should only include the internal luminal diameter. Portal vein (PV), inferior vena cava (IVC).

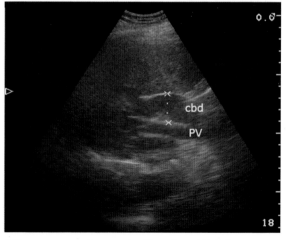

CBD measurement, accurate: The calipers (x's) indicate an internal luminal diameter of 2.5 cm.

63

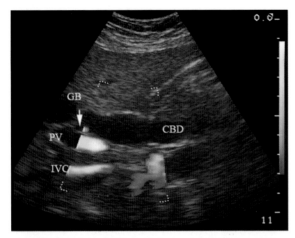

CBD dilation: Dilated CBD and "olive sandwich sign." The CBD measures 1.6 cm, significant for dilation, "sandwiching" the hepatic artery (arrow) – the "olive" – between the portal vein (PV).

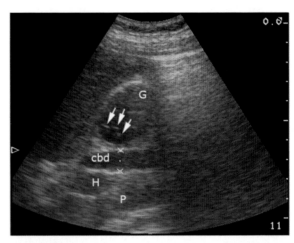

CBD dilation: The gallbladder (G) with three, non-shadowing stones (arrows). The cbd's internal diameter is appropriately measured (x's) to 1.1 cm, significant for dilation.

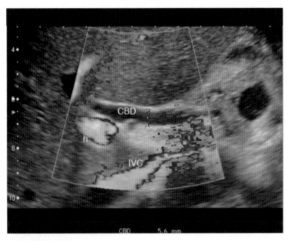

CBD dilation: cbd dilated to 5.6 mm overlying the hepatic artery (h) and IVC.

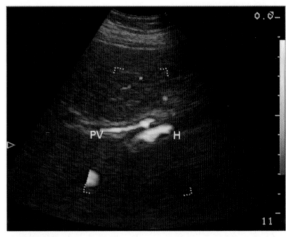

Fool's CBD: A dilated hepatic artery (H) posterior to the portal vein can mimic the CBD. Power Doppler demonstrates flow in both the portal vein (PV) and inferior vena cava, and therefore rules out either as being the CBD.

Ascites

Commonly encountered, ascites can disrupt accurate image interpretation. But an understanding of its characteristics can lead to clearly distinguishing its presence. Free fluid, like that of ascites, does not take an organized form, but instead "wedges" into spaces with sharp angles. Its anechoic nature attenuates imaging and can often improve images.

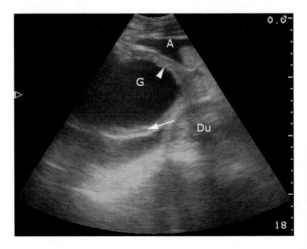

Classic ascites: In this case lying anteriorly, ascites (A) is seen bordered by the peritoneum anteriorly, thickened anterior gallbladder (G) wall posteriorly (arrowhead), and creating sharp, wedge-like angles around the adjacent bowel. Gallbladder (G), thickened gallbladder wall (arrow), duodenum (Du).

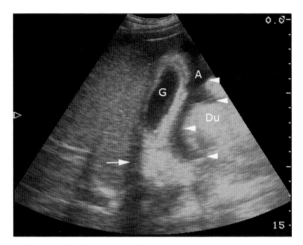

Classic ascites: Large fluid collection (A) inferior to the gallbladder (G) on longitudinal scan, outlining (arrowheads) the duodenum (Du) indicates ascites. Edge refraction shadowing (arrow).

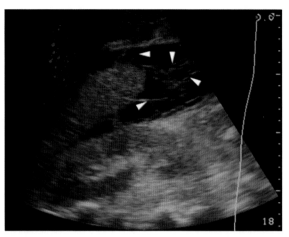

Loculated ascites: Multiple, wispy, hyperechoic septations (arrowheads) are visualized within this large, anechoic ascitic collection.

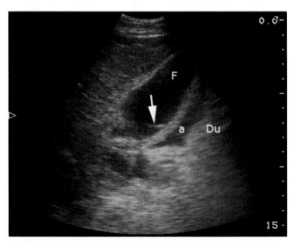

Undifferentiated free fluid: When lying posterior to the gallbladder, ascitic fluid (a) can be misinterpreted as pericholecystic fluid, but its proximity to the duodenum (Du), and characteristic wedging around the small bowel contours, helps clarify this as ascites. Gallbladder fundus (F), neck fold (arrow).

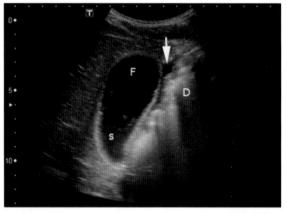

Undifferentiated free fluid: The small wedge of fluid (arrow) interspersed between gallbladder and duodenum (D) represents ascites and not PCF, as it tracks both anteriorly and posteriorly along the duodenal wall. Gallbladder fundus (F), sludge (s)).

Gallbladder wall thickening

An indicator of more severe pathology, the thickness of the gallbladder wall (GBW) should be noted and measured. A wall less than 0.3 cm in thickness is often considered normal.

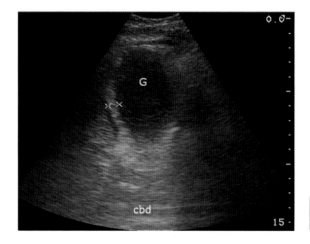

GBW thickening: Appropriately measured gallbladder (G) wall (x's) from the luminal outer wall to inner. Common bile duct (cbd).

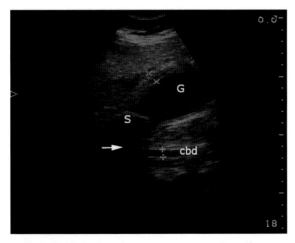

GBW thickening: An appropriately measured wall, significant for thickening, likely as a result of the large neck stone (s). Common bile duct (cbd), acoustic shadow (arrow).

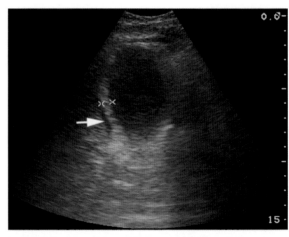

GBW thickening with pericholecystic fluid: A thickened GBW (x's) is seen outlined by a wedge-like, anechoic fluid collection which represents pericholecystic fluid (arrow).

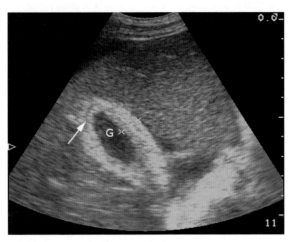

GBW thickening with pericholecystic fluid: A fine sliver of fluid (arrow) lies inferior to a thickened gallbladder wall (arrowhead). Gallbladder (G).

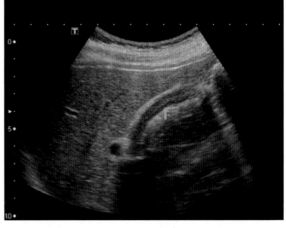

Contracted gallbladder: Often misinterpreted for pathologic gallbladder wall thickening, a hyperechoic wall of a contracted gallbladder (arrow).

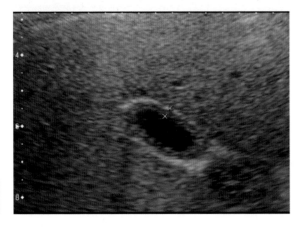

Contracted gallbladder: When magnified, a contracted gallbladder wall is more easily measured. In this case the patient had a recent meal and therefore the significance of this thickening is not relevant.

Pneumobilia

An indication of pathology, pneumobilia (or aerobilia) can often be identified on ultrasound as it accumulates in the biliary tree, and occasionally within the gallbladder wall. Pneumobilia casts distal reverberation artifact (comet-tailing) or shadowing which can often lead to its being misdiagnosed as a stone, a delineation that relies on location to elucidate.

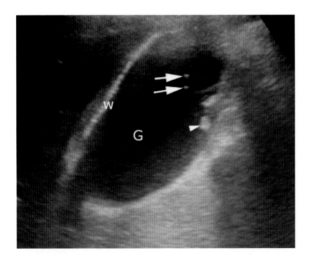

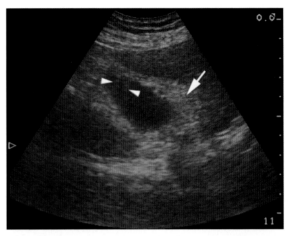

Pneumobilia, biliary tree: Air in the intrahepatic biliary ducts (arrows) is hyperechoic and casts a distal shadow (arrowhead).

Intraluminal air: Comet-tailing (arrowheads) extending from the gallbladder wall near the fundus is indicative of intraluminal air and significant illness. Thickened gallbladder wall (arrow).

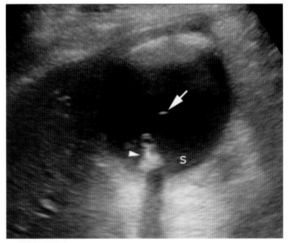

Air bubbles: Not all pneumobilia is confined to isolated locales, but can be seen ascending as hyperechoic circles (arrows) through the liquid medium of the gallbladder (G). Gallstone (arrowhead), wall inflammation (w).

Air bubbles: A single, non-shadowing, hyperechoic air bubble (arrow) ascends adjacent to a large stone (arrowhead). Biliary sludge (s).

Sludge

As particulate matter from bile precipitates – as a result of obstruction, medications, dietary changes, or otherwise – biliary sludge is the result. The increased viscosity of the sludge acts similarly to gallstones and can cause obstruction in the same manner, and therefore can be considered of equal significance to cholelithiasis in symptomatic patients.

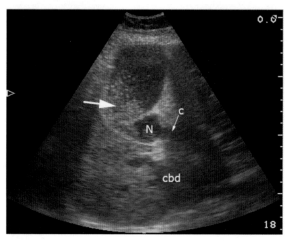

Sludge: Isoechoic in nature, sludge (arrow) often does not shadow, but will commonly layer along the most dependent aspects of the biliary tract, depending on its specific gravity. Neck (N), cystic duct (c), common bile duct (cbd).

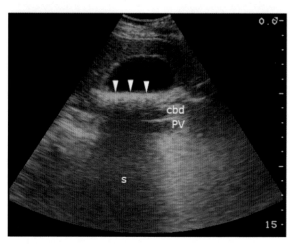

Shadowing sludge: The more particulate matter precipitated, the more sonographically obstructing sludge becomes (arrowheads) and can result in an acoustic shadow (s). Common bile duct (cbd), portal vein (PV).

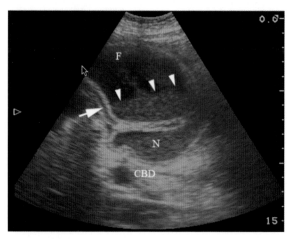

Severe sludge: Layering of sludge (arrowheads) within the gallbladder with signs of wall inflammation (arrow) and far-field acoustic attenuation. Fundus (F), neck (N), common bile duct (cbd).

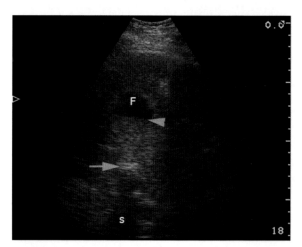

Sludge and stone: Sludge layering (arrowhead) posterior to the gallbladder fundus (F) overlying a large neck stone (arrow) demarcated by its marked hyperechoic rim and distal acoustic shadowing (s).

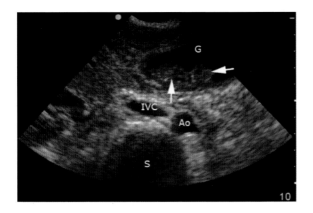

Biloma: As sludge thickens and congeals, it does not always precipitate a stone, but instead can form tumefactive sludge, or a biloma (arrows). This non-shadowing, heteroechoic, polypoid mass extending into the gallbladder (G) lumen must be distinguished from a neoplasm and often is found to be mobile when the patient is placed in the left lateral decubitus position, though biopsy is the only definitive diagnostic choice. Inferior vena cava (IVC), aorta (Ao), spine shadow (S).

Biliary polyps

Requiring further workup to rule out neoplasm, biliary polyps are a common pathology, occurring anywhere along the luminal wall, often non-shadowing, isoechoic structures that are immobile.

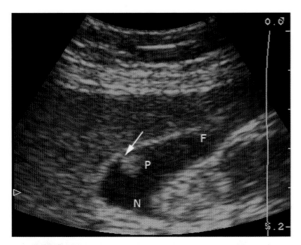

Biliary polyp: A polyp (P) and fine stalk (arrow) is attached to the anterior gallbladder wall, not to be confused with a stone which would likely orient in the dependent aspects of the gallbladder. Fundus (F), neck (N).

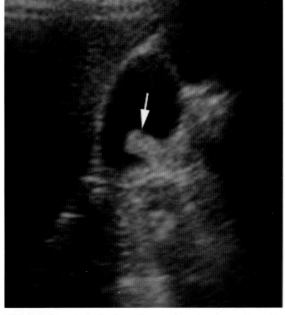

Biliary polyp: A single, dependent, pedunculated mass (arrow) is identified as a polyp because of its lack of acoustic shadowing and large affixing stalk.

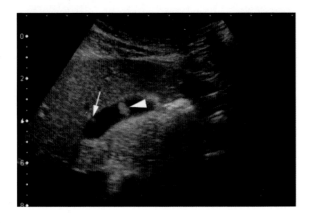

Polyposis: A small polyp (arrow), attached by a fine, hyperechoic insertive pedicle lies superior to a large, fixed mass (arrowhead) whose pedicle is not clearly seen (likely located on a lateral wall). Both are excluded as stones due to the lack of shadowing artifact.

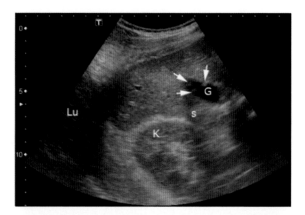

Polyposis: Multiple, small polyps (arrows) at the gallbladder (G) fundus, right lung (Lu), kidney (K).

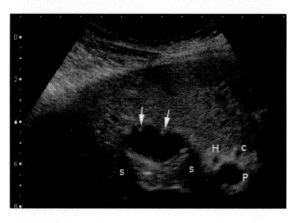

Polyposis: The finding of one polyp should prompt the search for others, although even a solitary polyp should prompt further diagnostic workup for possible neoplastic disease. Polyps (arrows), edge refraction artifact shadowing (s), hepatic artery (H), common bile duct (c), portal vein (P), the "Mickey Mouse sign."

WES sign

The "wall-echo-shadow" (WES) sign, or "double-arch" sign results from a contracted gallbladder around a large stone. The anterior-most hyperechoic line represents that of the gallbladder wall, with the second hyperechoic rim being that of the anterior crest of the stone. Interposed between the two layers is a hypoechoic brim of bile.

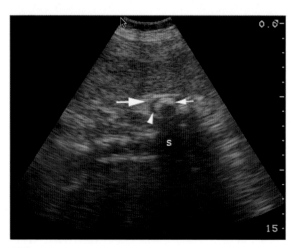

WES: The gallbladder wall (large arrow) overlies a hypoechoic wedge of bile or gallbladder lumen (arrowhead), encircling the hyperechoic gallstone brim (small arrow), which casts its distal acoustic shadow (s).

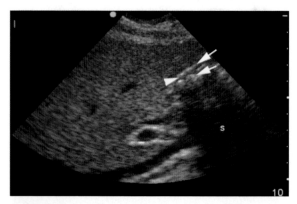

Difficult WES: Two hyperechoic rims (arrows) are seen sandwiching a hypoechoic region (arrowhead) and casting a far-field shadow (s).

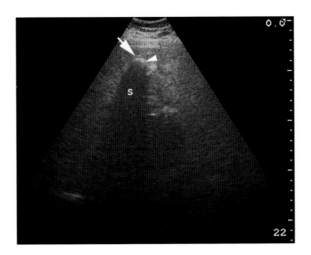

Good WES: In obese patients with poor acoustic windows, the WES's shadow (S) can be the only indicator as to the location of a contracted gallbladder (arrow) around a large stone (arrowhead).

Duodenum

Commonly misinterpreted as a gallbladder with multiple stones, the duodenum actually helps orient a sonographer to the location of the gallbladder. The duodenum is sonographically distinguished by its lack of distal field clarity as a result of duodenal air, which obscures the imaging. To further differentiate the duodenum from the gallbladder one can look for peristalsis, which should occur in the duodenum at regular intervals.

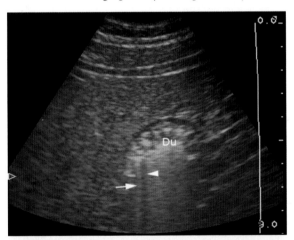

Duodenum: Resembling the classic "peas in a pod" appearance of a collection of gallstones, the duodenum (Du) is marked as being hyperechoic and having a mixture of comet-tailing (arrow) and distal acoustic shadowing (arrowhead) as a result of its mixed gaseous and particulate contents, respectively.

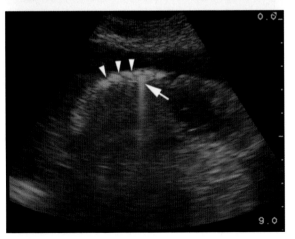

Duodenum: Another key feature distinguishing the duodenum from the gallbladder is the visualization of plicae circularae (arrowheads). Comet tail as a result of intestinal air (arrow).

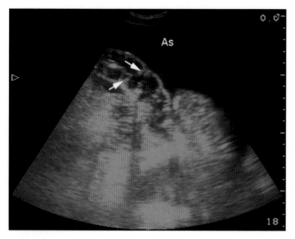

Duodenum: Outlined by a large collection of anechoic ascitic fluid (As), the plicae circularae (arrows) of the duodenum identify the structure as bowel.

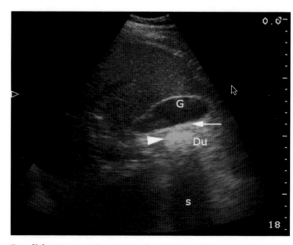

Fecalith: Commonly mistaken for a gallstone because of its echogenicity and distal shadowing (s), the duodenum (Du) can contain fecaliths (arrowhead), which can abut the gallbladder (G), but are clearly outside the gallbladder wall (arrow).

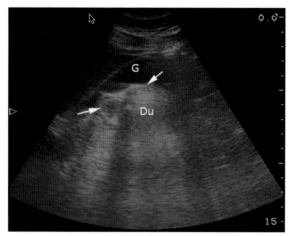

Fecalith: It is important to identify the posterior gallbladder (G) wall (arrows and note their continuity in overlying hyperechoic structures such as the duodenum (Du).

Liver pathology

Emergency bedside ultrasonography is not limited to the imaging of the gallbladder and biliary pathology, but can expand itself to the identification of numerous other forms of hepatic pathology.

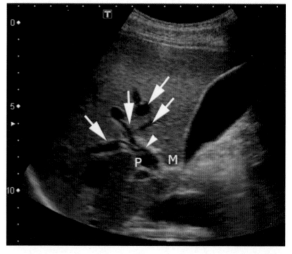

Dilated hepatic ducts: Indicative of possible biliary obstruction or chronic hepatic disease, dilated intrahepatic biliary ducts (arrows) are seen converging into the proximal bile duct confluence (arrowhead). Portal vein (P). Main lobar fissure (M).

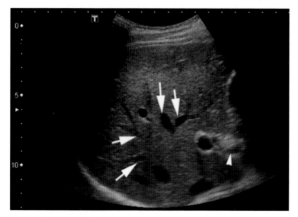

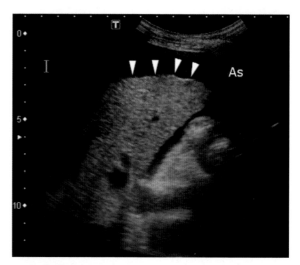

Dilated hepatic ducts: Sustained choledocholithiasis can cause resultant upstream generalized hepatic ductal dilation (arrows). Cystic duct (arrowhead).

Cirrhotic liver: The irregular, nodular edge of the liver (arrowheads) outlined by ascitic fluid (As) identifies a cirrhotic liver.

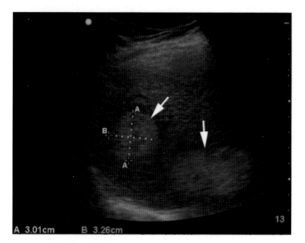

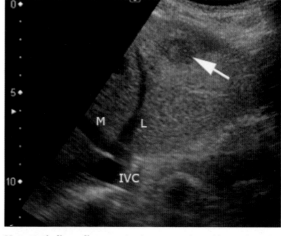

Metastatic liver disease: Two, well-circumscribed, heterogeneous and hypoechoic liver masses (arrows).

Metastatic liver disease: A solitary, coin-shaped lesion (arrow) likely represents neoplastic changes, but would require further studies to differentiate from benign processes such as hemangiomas. Middle hepatic vein (M), left hepatic vein (L), inferior vena cava (IVC).

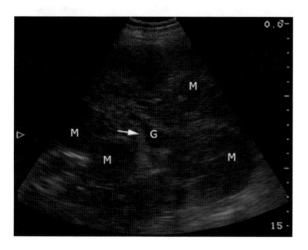

Metastatic liver disease: Multiple circular lesions (M) clearly represent metastatic disease, differentiated from the more anechoic gallbladder (G) with its anechoic lumen and well-defined wall (arrow).

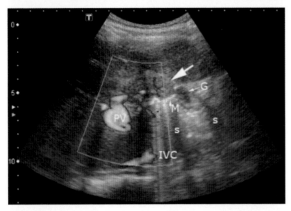

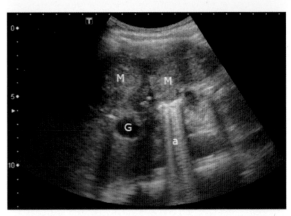

Metastatic liver disease: A heterogenous density (arrow) with evidence of central flow under power Doppler distinguishes this neoplastic mass from the gallbladder (G), seen casting two edge refraction shadows (s). Portal vein (PV), main lobar fissure (M), inferior vena cava (IVC).

Metastatic liver disease: Two heteroechoic, coin-shaped masses (M) identify liver metastases, one of which contains air, as indicated by its distal acoustic enhancement or "comet-tailing" (a). Gallbladder (G).

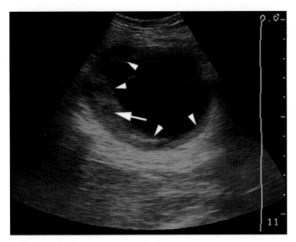

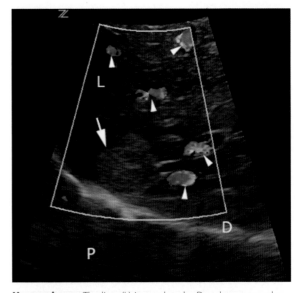

Cholangiocarcinoma: An echogenic, heterogenous mass (arrowheads) is seen invading the lumen of the gallbladder and contains hypoechoic irregularities (arrow). The diagnosis of cholangiocarcinoma was later confirmed after biopsy to distinguish it from a biloma.

Hemangioma: The liver (L) imaged under Doppler sonography shows multiple vascular structures (arrowheads) and a heterogenous, hyperechoic mass (arrow) indicative of a hemangioma. Diaphragm (D), right lung base (P).

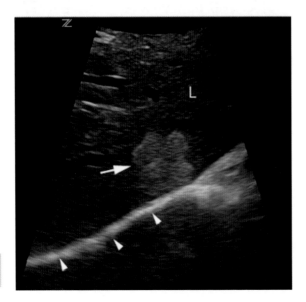

Hemangioma: A hyperechoic, heterogenic, nodular mass (arrow) abutting the diaphragm (arrowheads) within the liver (L) likely identifies a hemangioma.

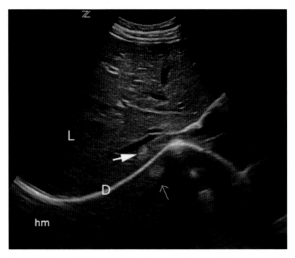

Hemangioma: A hyperechoic, heterogenic mass (heavy arrow) near the diaphragm (D) likely representing a hemangioma casts a mirror artifact into the chest (fine arrow). Liver (L).

Pleural effusion: Often the result of serious liver pathology, a pleural effusion (PE) can be identified in the lung by the absence of the normal mirror artifact across the diaphragm. The diaphragm (arrow) divides the heteroechoic liver (L) inferiorly from the hypoechoic fluid collection superiorly. Should an effusion or other abnormal substance collection not accumulate in the lung, the liver will reflect across the hyperechoic diaphragm, creating a mirror artifact. Liver mass (M).

Pancreas

An often unimaged, but usually easily identifiable structure adjacent to the readily imaged liver and gallbladder is the pancreas. Slightly more hyperechoic but equally as heterogenous as the liver, the pancreas can provide clues to biliary pathology. When more hyperechoic, it conveys underlying inflammation and possible outlet obstruction, imploring the sonographer to more carefully assess the biliary tree for dilation, thickening, stones, sludge, or other pathology. Moreover, the pancreas can occasionally present with pseudocysts, which sonographically are difficult to distinguish from the gallbladder when seen by novice sonographers.

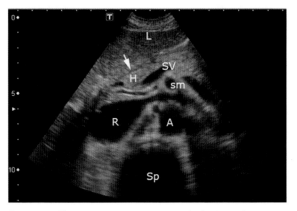

Anatomy: The superior mesenteric artery (sm) orients the sonographer to the location of the pancreas, seen "nutcracking" the left renal vein (R) overlying the aorta (A). Sitting atop the sm lies the splenic vein which posteriorly borders the body of the pancreas and identifies the pancreatic head (H), distinguished from the left lobe of the liver (L) by a fine, hypoechoic sliver (arrow). Spine shadow (Sp).

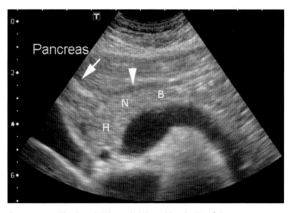

Anatomy: The head (H), neck (N) and body (B) of the pancreas are found immediately anterior to the hypoechoic, arching splenic vein. Occasionally, the pancreatic duct of Wirsung (arrowhead) can be seen adjoining to the common bile duct (arrow), an important point of interest for patients with elevated lipases and concern for gallstone pancreatitis.

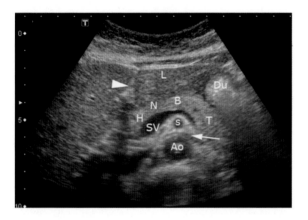

Anatomy: A sonographer interested in identifying the pancreas should first identify the aorta (Ao) and search for the superior mesenteric artery (S) lying in the same axis as the aorta, "nutcracking" the left renal vein (arrow) which lies posteriorly, and resting like a "mantle clock" beneath the splenic vein (SV). Anterior to the splenic vein sits the head (H), neck (N), body (B), and tail (T) of the pancreas, seen lying inferior to the left lobe of the liver (L), which tends to be of more hypoechoic, heterogenous composition than the pancreas. Falciform ligament (arrowhead). Duodenum (Du).

Intestinal ultrasound

Warren Wiechmann and Chase Warren

The appendix

Although it can be difficult to detect in its myriad positions around the cecum, locating the appendix and determining whether it is normal or inflamed is a rapid and cost-effective way of ruling out or making a diagnosis of appendicitis. This is determined by measuring the diameter, compressibility, and power Doppler data obtained from the ultrasound scan.

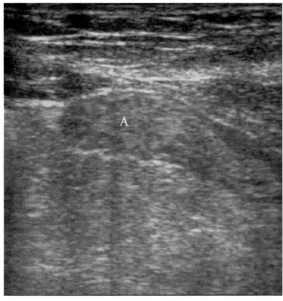

Normal appendix, long axis: Long-axis view of a normal appendix, which is often quite elusive and difficult to even detect. When observed, it presents as a compressible tube that is 5 mm or less in diameter.

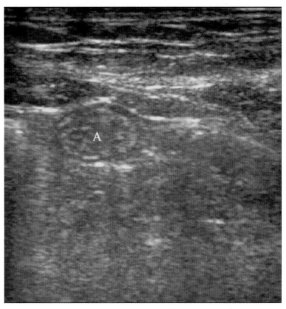

Normal appendix, short axis: Short-axis view of a normal appendix (A), which is often quite elusive and difficult to detect. When observed, it presents as a compressible tube that is 5 mm or less in diameter.

Atlas of Emergency Ultrasound, ed. John Christian Fox. Published by Cambridge University Press. © J.C. Fox 2011.

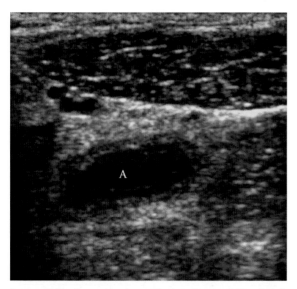

Appendicitis, long axis: Long-axis view of appendicitis, which is an inflamed appendix (A) > 6 mm in diameter, non-compressible, and filled with hypoechoic fluid infiltrate.

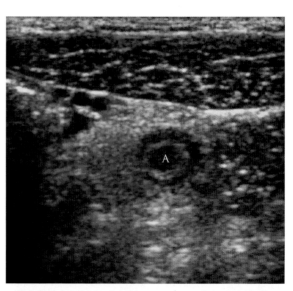

Appendicitis, short axis: Short-axis view of appendicitis, which is an inflamed appendix (A) > 6 mm in diameter, non-compressible, and filled with hypoechoic fluid infiltrate.

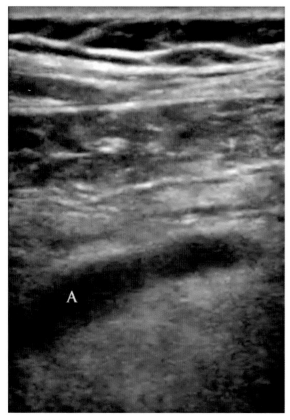

Appendicitis, long axis: Long-axis view of appendicitis, which is an inflamed appendix (A) > 6 mm in diameter, non-compressible, and filled with hypoechoic fluid infiltrate.

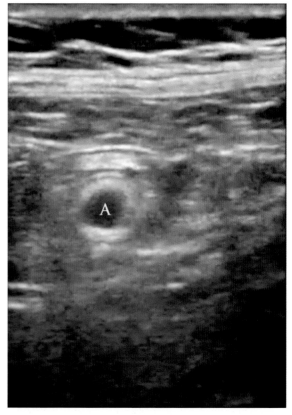

Appendicitis short axis: Short-axis view of appendicitis, which is an inflamed appendix (A) > 6 mm in diameter, non-compressible, and filled with hypoechoic fluid infiltrate.

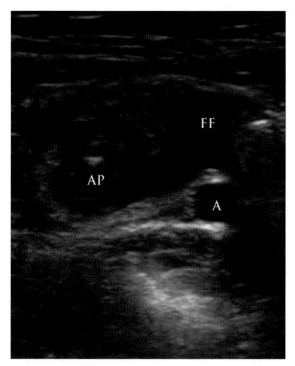

Periappendiceal free fluid: In acute appendicitis, hypoechoic free fluid (FF) can accumulate in the space directly surrounding the inflamed appendix (AP). Artery (A).

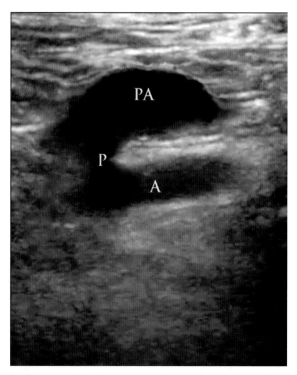

Perforated appendix: In a long-axis view of acute appendicitis, a perforation (P) can form in the appendiceal tissue, allowing the hypoechoic fluid contents of the inflamed appendix (A) to escape and create an abscess (PA) in nearby tissue.

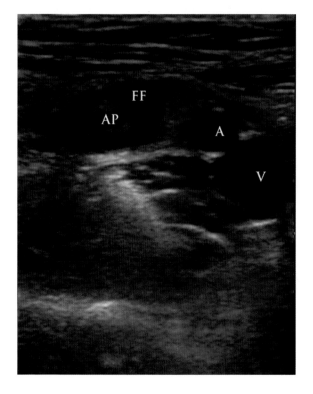

Periappendiceal free fluid: In acute appendicitis, hypoechoic free fluid (FF) can accumulate in the space directly surrounding the inflamed appendix (AP). Artery (A), vein (V).

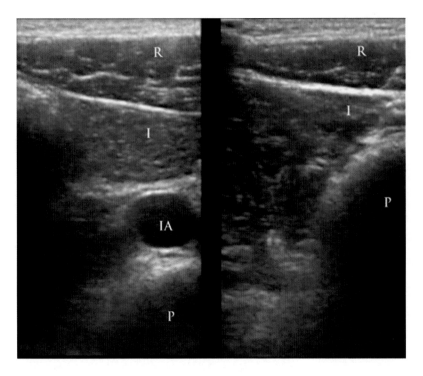

Psoas rectus compression: When the transducer head is firmly pressed against the abdomen, the rectus (R) muscle should be able to come into direct contact with the psoas (P) muscle. In the case of appendicitis, the inflamed and non-compressible appendix prohibits this from occurring, and a gap between the two muscles is felt and observed. Intestine (I), iliac artery (IA).

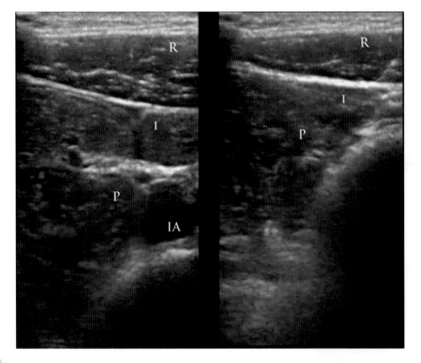

Psoas rectus compression: When the transducer head is firmly pressed against the abdomen, the rectus (R) muscle should be able to come into direct contact with the psoas (P) muscle. In the case of appendicitis, the inflamed and non-compressible appendix prohibits this from occurring, and a gap between the two muscles is felt and observed. Intestine (I), iliac artery (IA).

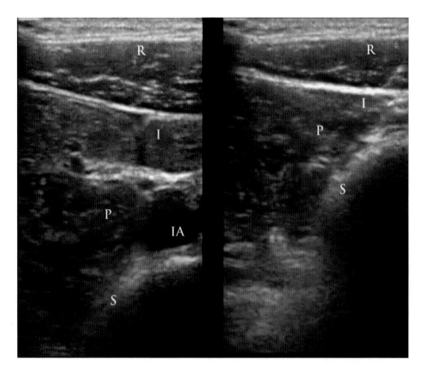

Psoas rectus compression, long-axis view: When the transducer head is firmly pressed against the abdomen, the rectus (R) muscle should be able to come into direct contact with the psoas (P) muscle. In the case of appendicitis, the inflamed and non-compressible appendix prohibits this from occurring, and a gap between the two muscles is felt and observed. Intestine (I), iliac artery (IA), sacrum (S).

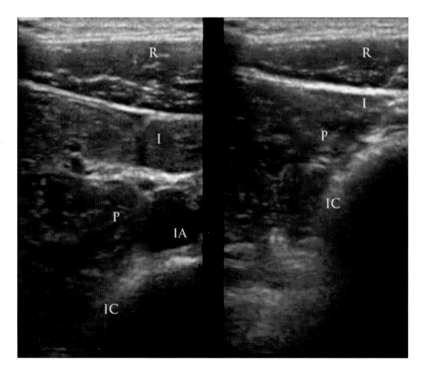

Psoas rectus compression, short-axis view: When the transducer head is firmly pressed against the abdomen, the rectus (R) muscle should be able to come into direct contact with the psoas (P) muscle. In the case of appendicitis, the inflamed and non-compressible appendix prohibits this from occurring, and a gap between the two muscles is felt and observed. Intestine (I), iliac artery (IA), iliac crest (IC).

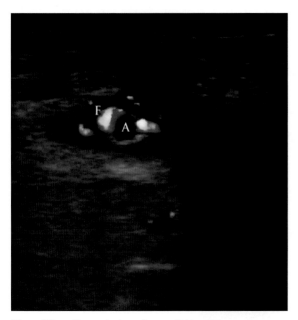

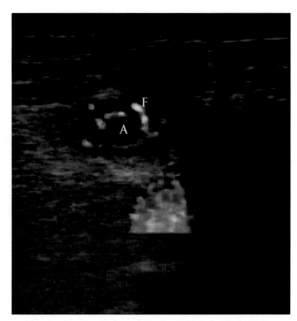

Ring of fire: Short-axis view of appendicitis utilizing power Doppler, which creates a distinct "ring of fire" (F) appearance around the appendix (A) in response to the increased blood flow to the inflamed area.

Ring of fire: Short-axis view of appendicitis utilizing power Doppler, which creates a distinct "ring of fire" (F) appearance around the appendix (A) in response to the increased blood flow to the inflamed area. The second "flame" is artifact.

Ascites

Free fluid in the abdominal cavity is an important etiology to prove when assessing abdominal distension and pain, and an absolutely crucial finding when incidentally noted during an unrelated scan.

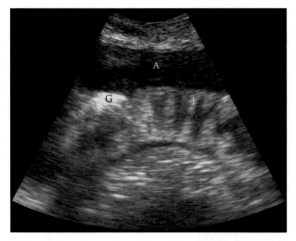

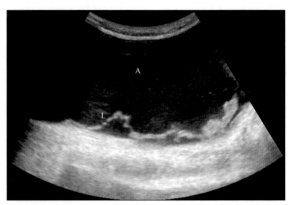

Abdominal ascites and small bowel peristalsis: A portion of the small intestine (I) undergoing a peristaltic contraction (note the compressed plicae circulares) adjacent to the hypoechoic abdominal ascites fluid (A). Intestinal gas (G) shows as a hyperechoic mass along the edge of the intestine.

Loculations: Loculations (L) (wispy, cobweb-like filaments) within the hypoechoic abdominal ascites fluid (A), that undulate and ripple with movement.

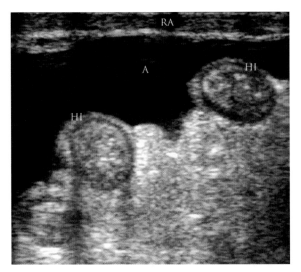

Ascites surrounding small bowel short axis: Cross-sectional view of small intestine loops (HI) peristalsing, adjacent to the hypoechoic abdominal ascites fluid (A). Rectus abdominis (RA).

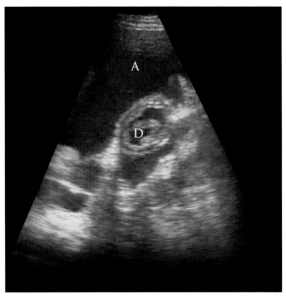

Duodenum surrounded by ascites: Short-axis view of a duodenum (D) segment surrounded by hypoechoic ascites fluid (A).

Diverticulitis

Diverticuli, havens for fecaliths and food matter, are vital to identify when evaluating patients with localized left lower quadrant pain, fever, and leukocytosis.

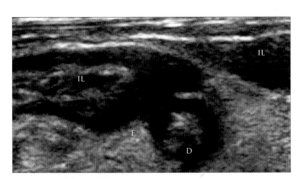

Diverticulitis: Diverticulum (D), which is an outward finger-like projection of intestinal lumen (IL). Often, it is surrounded by fat (F) and a thickened, edematous intestinal wall.

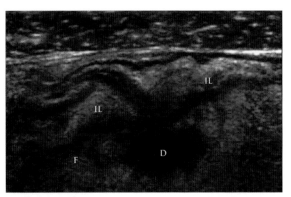

Diverticulitis: Diverticulum (D), which is an outward finger-like projection of intestinal lumen (IL). Often, it is surrounded by fat (F) and a thickened, edematous intestinal wall.

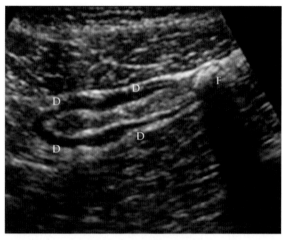

Fecalith within diverticulitis, long axis: Long-axis view of a fecalith (F), entrapped and hardened fecal matter within a diverticulum (D) of the intestine. Note the shadow the fecalith casts.

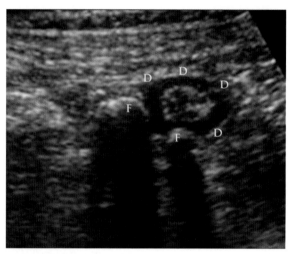

Fecalith within diverticulitis short axis: Short-axis view of a fecalith (F), entrapped and hardened fecal matter within a diverticulum (D) of the intestine. Note the shadow the fecaliths casts.

Hernia

Ultrasound offers a modality unique from the other imaging sources such as CT and films, allowing hernias to be viewed not only statically but in motion and in real time. The extent of protrusion and nature of the defective body wall can be accurately described and measured.

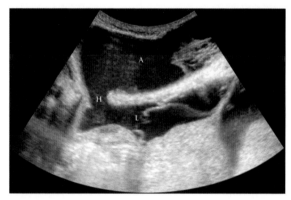

Ventral hernia with ascites and loculations: Loculations (L) (wispy, cobweb-like filaments) within the hypoechoic abdominal ascites fluid (A). A ventral wall defect (H) is present, with a significant amount of ascites outside and within the hernia itself.

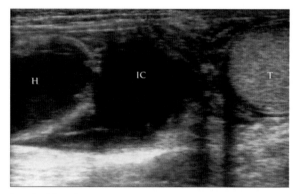

Inguinal hernia: Herniated intestine (I) protruding into and descending along the inguinal canal (IC) toward the testicle (T).

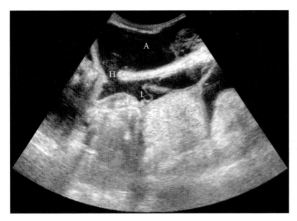

Hernia, ascites, and loculations: Loculations (L) (wispy, cobweb-like filaments) within the hypoechoic abdominal ascites fluid (A). A ventral wall defect (H) is present, with a significant amount of ascites outside and within the hernia itself.

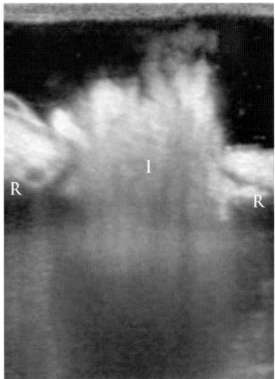

Umbilical hernia: Herniated loop of intestine (I) breaching the rectus abdominis (R) in the umbilical region of the abdomen, surrounded by hypoechoic ascites fluid.

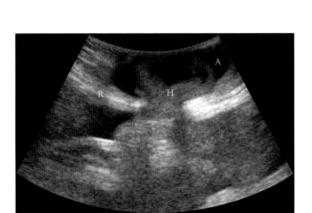

Ventral hernia: Herniated loop of intestine (H) breaching the rectus abdominis (R), surrounded by hypoechoic abdominal ascites fluid (A).

Intussusception

Especially prevalent in children, intussusception is the inversion of bowel back within itself. Ultrasound is both specific and highly sensitive in detecting the close concentric layers of bowel wall that are pathognomonic of the disease.

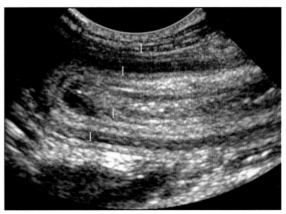

Intussusception, long axis: Long-axis view of an intussusception (I), wherein a segment of bowel is pushed retrograde into the segment of bowel preceding it. This forms concentric layers of bowel, similar to a collapsible telescope.

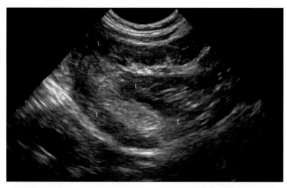

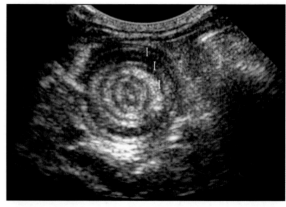

Intussusception, long axis pseudo-kidney sign: The telescoping bowel segments of an Intussusception bend to form a kidney-like shape in the long-axis view. Bowel lumen (L).

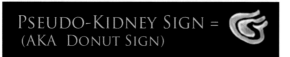

Intussusception, short axis: Short-axis view of an intussusception (I), wherein a segment of bowel is pushed retrograde into the segment of bowel preceding it. This forms concentric layers of bowel, similar to a collapsible telescope.

Small bowel obstruction

Easily confused with ileus, obstruction of the small intestine can present ultrasonically with free fluid between intestinal loops and an increased thickness of the bowel wall.

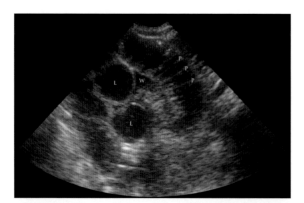

Small bowel obstruction: Short-axis view of obstructed small intestine. The increased pressure within the obstructed bowel forces fluid outward through the strained intestinal wall into the abdominal cavity, creating free fluid wedges (W). Trapped fecal matter (F) can be seen languishing in the bowel loops (L).

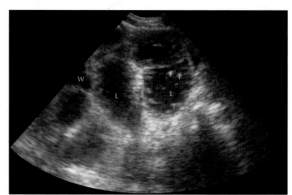

Small bowel obstruction: Short-axis view of obstructed small intestine. The increased pressure within the obstructed bowel forces fluid outward through the strained intestinal wall into the abdominal cavity, creating free fluid wedges (W). Trapped fecal matter (F) can be seen languishing in the bowel loops (L).

Odds and ends

Although unanimously claimed as accidental but almost always intentional, events of a "delicate nature" can benefit greatly from a discreet ultrasound survey to assess extent and possible damage.

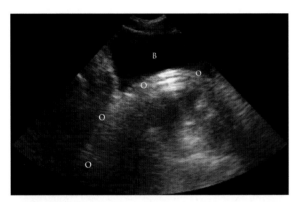

Rectal foreign body: Cross-sectional view of a 16 oz. bottle (O) completely filling the rectum and pushing against the urinary bladder (B).

Chapter 7

Pelvic ultrasound

Cindy Chau and John Christian Fox

Anatomy

The female internal organs are situated in the pelvic cavity. The size of the uterus varies at different ages and parities. A nulliparous adult uterus measures 6–8 cm in length versus 9–10 cm in multiparous women. The endometrial thickness also varies greatly in thickness, 0.5–5 mm. The ovaries can be difficult to identify. A normal size ovary measures about 3.5 × 2 × 1.5 cm and 1.5 × 0.7 × 0.5 cm in pre-menopausal and postmenopausal women, respectively. The uterus and pelvic vessels are used as landmarks for identifying the ovaries.

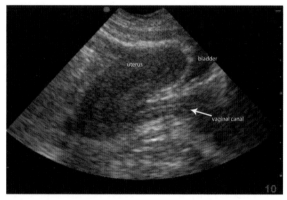

Transabdominal sonogram: Sagittal view of uterus.

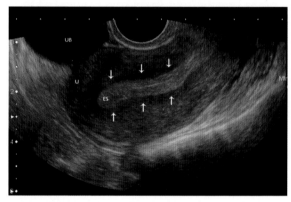

Transvaginal sonogram: Sagittal view. Endometrial stripe (ES, arrows), uterus (U), urinary bladder (UB).

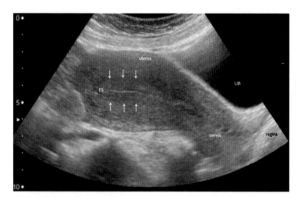

Transabdominal sonogram: Sagittal view. Endometrial stripe (ES, arrows), urinary bladder (UB).

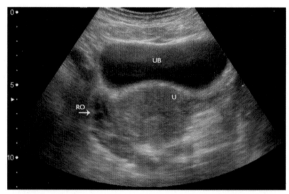

Transabdominal sonogram: Coronal view. Uterus (U), right ovary (RO) with multiple follicles, urinary bladder (UB).

Atlas of Emergency Ultrasound, ed. John Christian Fox. Published by Cambridge University Press. © J.C. Fox 2011.

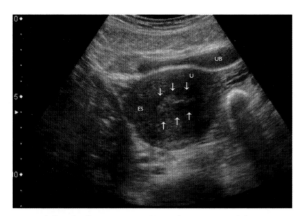

Transabdominal sonogram: Coronal view. Uterus (U), endometrial strip (ES, arrows), urinary bladder (UB).

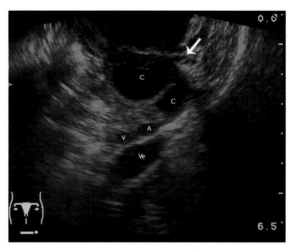

Ovaries: Transvaginal sonogram. Coronal oblique view. Left ovary (arrow) with multiple cysts (C), internal iliac artery (A) and vein (V), and external iliac vein (Ve). The ovaries lie anterior to the iliac vessels.

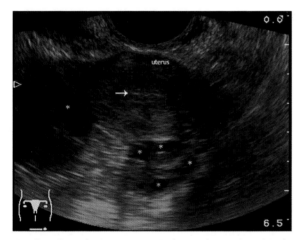

Ovaries: Coronal view sonogram. Endometrial stripe (arrow), right and left ovaries with multiple follicles (*). In this view, ovaries are located behind the uterus, posterior cul-de-sac, or pouch of Douglas.

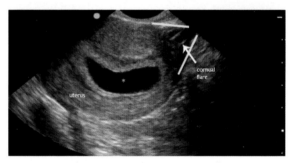

Pregnancy, abnormal: Coronal view sonogram: Abnormal pregnancy with pseudosac in utero (*). The "cornual flare," portion of the uterus at the junction of the fallopian tubes, aids in locating the ovaries and fallopian tubes via laterally moving the probe.

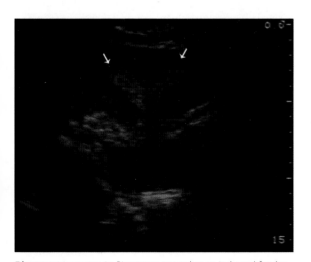

Bicornuate uterus 1: Bicornuate uterus has an indented fundus and two endometrial cavities (arrows) versus a septate uterus which has a normal external surface and two endometrial cavities.

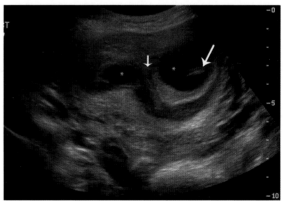

Bicornuate uterus 2: Pregnancy in a septate uterus: Note the normal external surface with two endometrial cavities (*). Septum (arrow). Intrauterine pregnancy in one horn – fetal pole (large arrow).

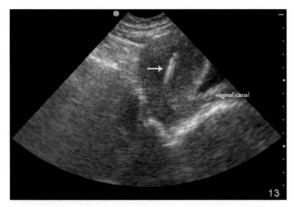

Intrauterine device: Transabdominal sonogram. Longitudinal plane. Intrauterine device (arrow).

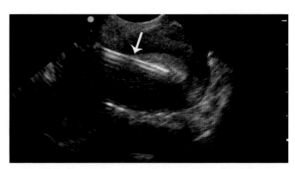

Intrauterine device: Transvaginal sonogram. Intrauterine device (arrow).

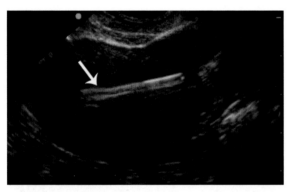

Intrauterine device: Transvaginal sonogram. Sagittal view. Intrauterine device.

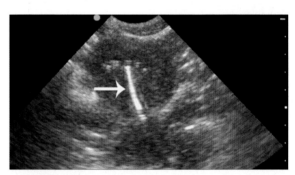

Intrauterine device: Transabdominal sonogram. Copper intrauterine device.

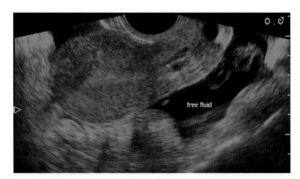

Free fluid: Transabdominal sonogram. Longitudinal plane. Patient with a ruptured ectopic pregnancy (not seen in this view). Note the empty uterus and free fluid in the pelvic cul-de-sac.

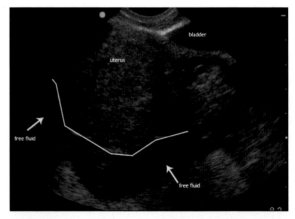

Free fluid: Coronal view sonogram. Ectopic pregnancy with free fluid in the pelvic cul-de-sac (pouch of Douglas). Free fluid may also be visualized in the hepatorenal recess. Free fluid is anechoic (black).

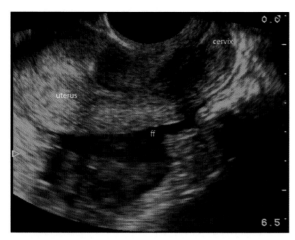

Free fluid: Transvaginal sonogram. Sagittal view. Free fluid (ff) in cul-de-sac. Note the heterogenicity of the fluid, likely clotted blood.

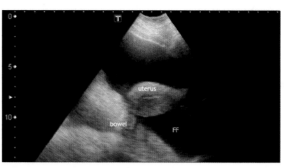

Free fluid: Transabdominal sonogram. Sagittal view. Free fluid (ff) in pelvic cul-de-sac (pouch of Douglas).

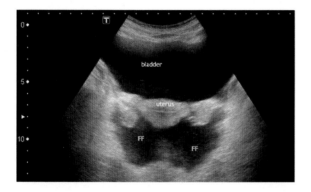

Free fluid: Transabdominal sonogram. Coronal view. Free fluid (ff) in pelvic cul-de-sac (pouch of Douglas).

Intrauterine pregnancy

The ability to visualize an intrauterine pregnancy (IUP) via sonography correlates with the level of beta-human chorionic gonadotropin (hCG). On transvaginal ultrasound examination, a gestational sac is visible at 4.5–5 weeks of gestation, which corresponds to an hCG level of > 1500 IU/L. The yolk sac appears between 5–6 weeks. A fetal pole is detectable at 5.5–6 weeks. Cardiac motion is detectable at hCG > 6000 IU/L. An IUP is visible via transabdominal ultrasound at >6500 IU/L.

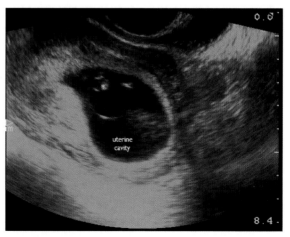

Intrauterine pregnancy: Transvaginal sonogram. Coronal view. Intrauterine pregnancy, fetal pole (*).

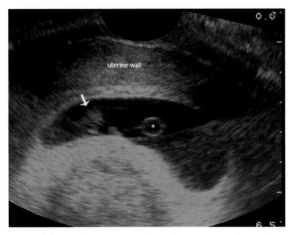

Intrauterine pregnancy: Transvaginal sonogram. Early intrauterine pregnancy. Presence of both yolk sac (*) and fetal pole (arrow) gives an estimated gestational age of 5–6 weeks.

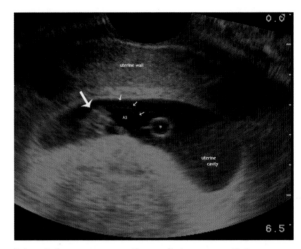

Intrauterine pregnancy: Transvaginal sonogram. Early intrauterine pregnancy. Presence of yolk sac (*), fetal pole (big arrow), and amniotic sac (small arrows, AS) gives an estimated gestational age of 5–6 weeks.

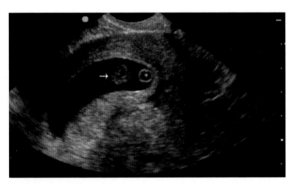

Intrauterine pregnancy: Coronal view sonogram. Early intrauterine pregnancy (IUP). Presence of fetal pole (arrow) and yolk sac (*) indicates a 5–6 week IUP.

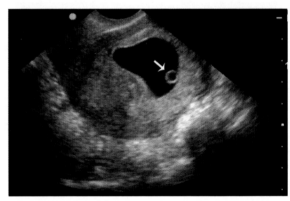

Intrauterine pregnancy: Transvaginal sonogram. Yolk sac (arrow) presence indicates a pregnancy at ~5 weeks gestational age.

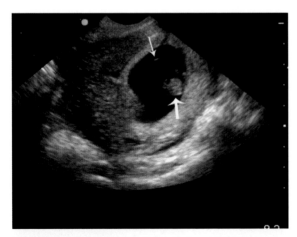

Intrauterine pregnancy: Transvaginal sonogram. Early intrauterine pregnancy, 6 weeks gestational age. Fetal pole (white arrow), yolk sac (not shown here), and amniotic sac (part of the amniotic sac membrane in yellow arrow).

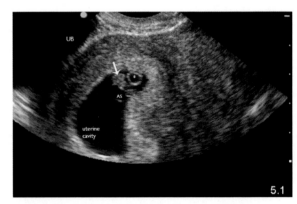

Intrauterine pregnancy: Transvaginal sonogram. Early intrauterine pregnancy, 6 weeks gestational age. A 2- to 3-mm gestational sac, yolk sac, and embryonic pole with cardiac activity are visualized via transvaginal ultrasound at gestational ages 4, 5, 6 weeks. Yolk sac (*), amniotic sac (AS), fetal pole (arrow), urinary bladder (UB).

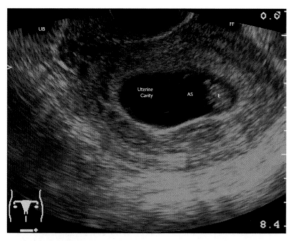

Intrauterine pregnancy: Transvaginal sonogram. Intrauterine pregnancy. Amniotic sac (AS), embryo (E), free fluid (ff), urinary bladder (UB).

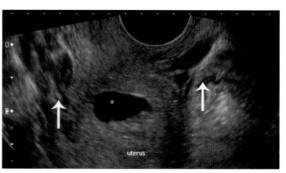

Intrauterine versus ectopic pregnancy: Transvaginal sonogram. Coronal view. Note empty intrauterine cavity. Early intrauterine pregnancy (IUP) versus ectopic pregnancy. Need to correlate with serum beta-hCG levels. Normal IUP is visible at beta-hCG 1500–2000 IU/L via transvaginal ultrasound and >6500 IU/L via transabdominal ultrasound. Bilateral ovaries with follicles (arrows).

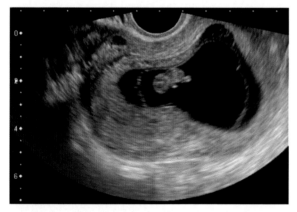

Intrauterine pregnancy, abnormal: Sonogram showing an abnormal intrauterine pregnancy with fetal demise. Note the collapsing and abnormally shaped gestational sac.

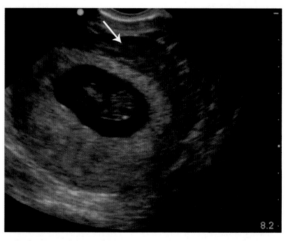

Subchorionic hemorrhage: First trimester subchorionic hemorrhage (arrow). Hematoma is collected between the uterine wall and the chorionic membrane. Vaginal bleeding may or may not be present. Patients are at increased risk of miscarriage, stillbirth, placental abruption, and preterm labor.

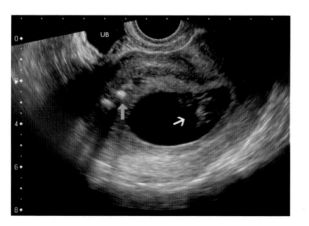

Intrauterine pregnancy with intrauterine device: Embryo (white arrow) and IUD (orange arrow). Urinary bladder (UB). Overall incidence of ectopic pregnancy is lower than the general population given its effectiveness in preventing pregnancies. However, patients are at increased risk of having an ectopic pregnancy if pregnancy occurs.

Ectopic pregnancy

Ectopic pregnancy is a pregnancy outside of the uterine cavity. The most common extra-uterine location is the fallopian tube (98%). Diagnostics tests include transvaginal ultrasound (TVUS) and quantitative beta-hCG. Absence of an IUP via TVUS at beta-hCG above the discriminatory zone, the level of hCG (>1500 IU/L) in which an IUP should be visualized by TVUS, increases the suspicion of an ectopic or nonviable intrauterine pregnancy. Color Doppler can be used to identify a "ring of fire" surrounding an ectopic pregnancy. A pseudosac, present in ~20%, of ectopic pregnancies, is a small fluid collection located within the endometrial cavity.

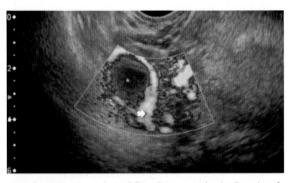

Ectopic pregnancy, ring of fire: Transvaginal color Doppler of adnexa showing the ring of fire (arrow), produced by the placental blood flow within the periphery of the complex adnexal mass. Ectopic pregnancy with a fetal pole (*).

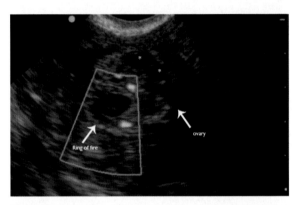

Ring of fire: The ring of fire is associated with ectopic pregnancies. Notice the adjacent ovary with follicles (*).

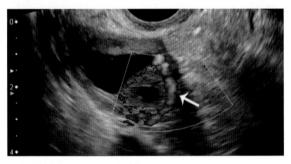

Ectopic pregnancy: Ring of fire.

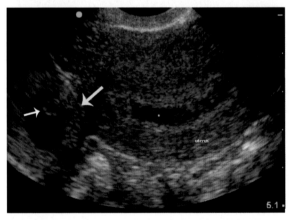

Ectopic pregnancy: Coronal view sonogram showing a right ectopic pregnancy. Note the gestational sac (yellow arrow) and yolk sac (white arrow). Uterine cavity with a pseudosac (*).

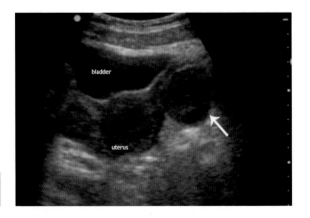

Ectopic pregnancy, cornuate versus tubal pregnancy: Transvaginal sonogram. Coronal view. Note the left sided cornuate versus tubal pregnancy (arrow).

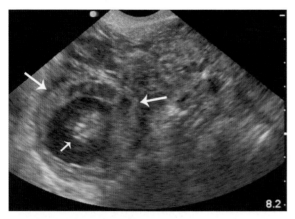

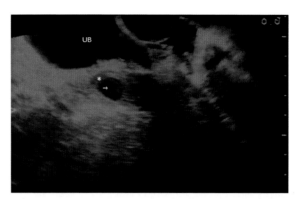

Ectopic pregnancy (cornual): The arrows outline a mass right along the edge of the uterus instead of in the fundus of the uterus. At this location, the edge of the uterus, the mantle is very thin and at risk for uterine rupture should the ectopic grow large enough. This is also termed "interstitial ectopic" as the pregnancy is located in the interstitium, the site at which the fallopian tube enters the uterus.

Ectopic pregnancy with pseudosac: Ectopic pregnancy with gestational sac (*) and fetal pole (arrow). Urinary bladder (UB). Uterine cavity with pseudosac (not shown here).

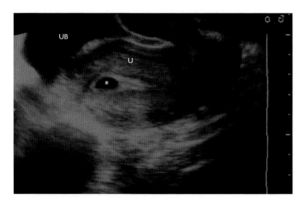

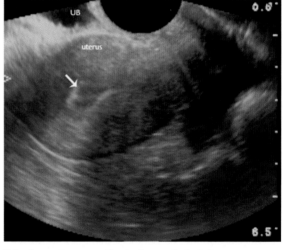

Ectopic pregnancy with pseudosac: Ectopic pregnancy (not shown here). Pseudosac (*) in the uterine cavity. Note the absence of the yolk sac and fetal pole. Uterus (U), urinary bladder (UB).

Ectopic pregnancy and pseudosac: Sagittal view sonogram. Ectopic pregnancy (not shown here) with intrauterine pseudosac (arrow). Note also the free fluid. Urinary bladder (UB).

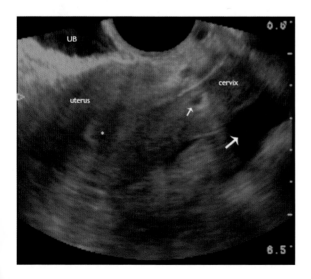

Ectopic pregnancy and free fluid: Sagittal view sonogram of patient with an ectopic pregnancy (not shown here). Nabothian cysts (small arrows). Free fluid (big arrow). Pseudosac (*), urinary bladder (UB).

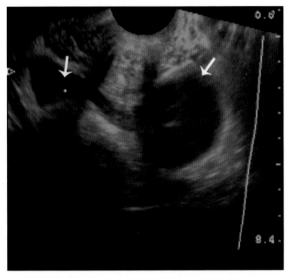

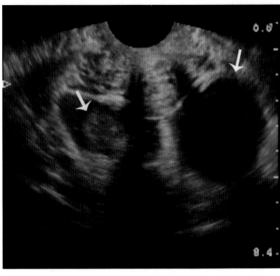

Ectopic pregnancy and free fluid: Coronal view sonogram. Patient with an ectopic pregnancy (yellow arrow), fetal pole (*, better viewed on another slide) and a hemorrhagic cyst (white arrow). Note the reticular/weblike pattern within the cyst.

Ectopic pregnancy and hemorrhagic cyst: Ectopic pregnancy, fetal pole (yellow arrow). Hemorrhagic ovarian cyst (white arrow).

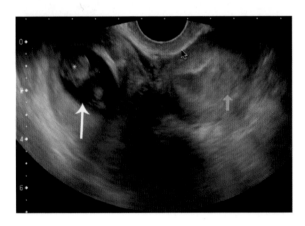

Ectopic pregnancy: Transabdominal sonogram. Ectopic pregnancy (white arrow). Embryo (*). Uterus (yellow arrow).

Molar pregnancy

Molar pregnancies, complete or partial mole, result from aberrant fertilization. Women typically present with signs and symptoms of early pregnancy. Some of the clinical manifestations include vaginal bleeding, enlarged uterus, pelvic pressure or pain, theca lutein cysts, anemia, hyperemesis gravidarum, hyperthyroidism, preeclampsia before 20 weeks of gestation and vaginal passage of hydropic vesicles.

Diagnostic evaluation includes quantitative beta-hCG and ultrasound. Beta-hCG levels are typically elevated, 40% greater than 100,000 IU/L. Ultrasound findings in a complete mole include absence of an embryo or fetus, no amniotic fluid, heterogenous mass with discrete anechoic spaces (corresponding to hydropic chorionic villi – described as snowstorm pattern).

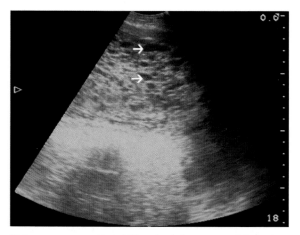

Molar pregnancy: Hydatidiform (molar) pregnancy: Echogenic mass in the uterine cavity with multiple small, hypoechoic areas (arrows).

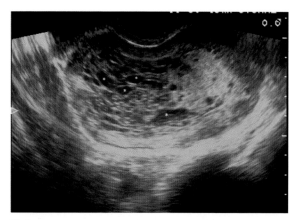

Molar pregnancy: Hydatidiform (molar) pregnancy. Echogenic mass with multiple hypoechoic areas (*) filling the uterine cavity. Note the "snow storm" effect on the sonogram.

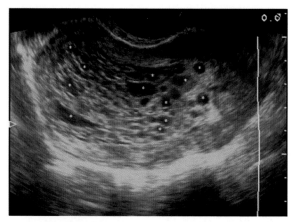

Molar pregnancy: Hydatidiform (molar) pregnancy. Echogenic mass filling the uterine cavity with multiple hypoechoic areas (*). Note the "snow storm" effect on the sonogram.

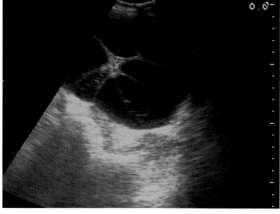

Molar pregnancy: Theca-lutein cysts, frequently seen in disorders with increased hCG such as multiple pregnancies, hydatidiform pregnancy (which this sonogram is derived from), choriocarcinoma, fetal hydrops, exogenous hCG treatment, or polycystic ovary. Typically, it has a multiloculated appearance.

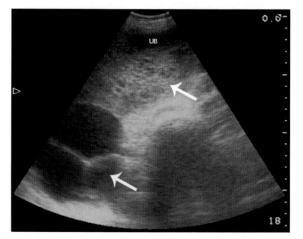

Molar pregnancy: Coronal view sonogram. Hydatidiform (molar) pregnancy (white arrow) and theca lutein cysts (yellow arrow). Note the echogenic mass with the hypoechoic areas filling the uterine cavity, and the typical multiloculated appearance in the right ovarian cysts. Urinary bladder (UB).

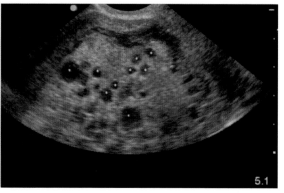

Molar pregnancy: Hydatidiform (molar) pregnancy: note the echogenic mass in the uterine cavity with multiple hypoechoic areas (*) secondary to trophoblastic proliferation and edema of villous stroma.

Cysts

Cysts are small fluid-filled sacs. There are different types of ovarian functional cysts: follicular (75% of all cysts), corpus luteum, hemorrhagic, dermoid, theca-lutein (bilateral) endometrioid, and polycystic-appearing ovaries. The internal cystic structure may be categorized into simple, complex or completely solid. When cysts are less than 6 cm in size in reproductive age women, management is to observe for 6–8 weeks plus a repeat ultrasound. Cysts are measured from outer wall to inner wall. When filled with blood or blood clots, cysts have a reticular or web-like pattern.

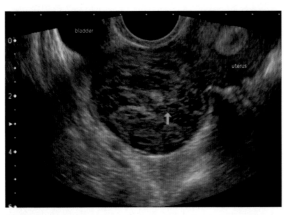

Ovarian mass: Transabdominal sonogram. Ovarian mass (arrow).

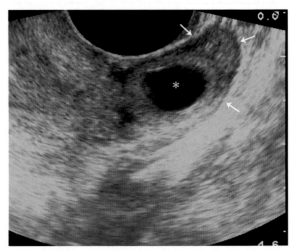

Corpus luteal cyst: Ovary (arrows), corpus luteal cyst (*). Viable intrauterine pregnancy (not shown here).

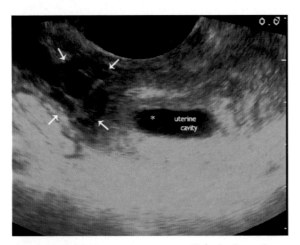

Ovarian follicles: Intrauterine pregnancy (*), fetal pole not shown here. Right ovary (arrows) with multiple follicles.

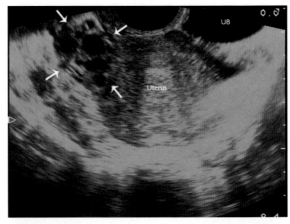

Ovarian follicles: Right ovary with multiple follicles (arrows). Urinary bladder (UB).

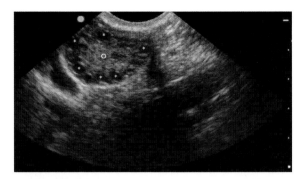

Ovaries: Multifollicular ovary (O), follicles (*).

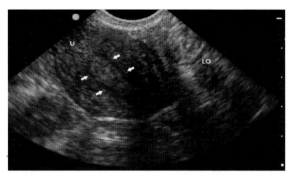

Ovaries: Transverse view. Left ovary (LO), endometrial stripe (arrows). Uterus (U).

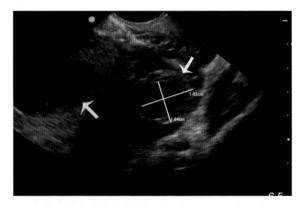

Corpus luteal cyst and IUP: Corpus luteal cyst (white arrow) and intrauterine pregnancy (yellow arrow; yolk sac and fetal pole not shown here). Cysts are measured from outer wall to inner wall, 1.64 × 1.82 cm.

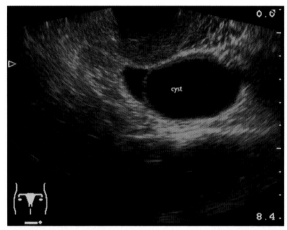

Ovarian cysts: Ovarian cyst.

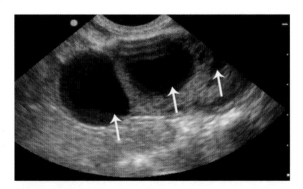

Ovarian cysts: Ovary with multiple simple cysts.

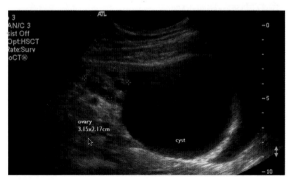

Ovarian cyst: Ovarian masses or cysts > 4 cm are at increased risk of torsion.

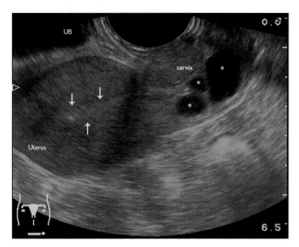

Nabothian cysts: Sagittal view. Nabothian cysts (*), located in the cervix. Normal appearing uterus with thin endometrial stripe (arrows). Urinary bladder (UB).

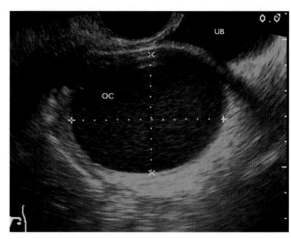

Hemorrhagic cyst: Left ovarian hemorrhagic cyst, 4 × 5 cm (OC), also known as a hematocele. Urinary bladder (UB).

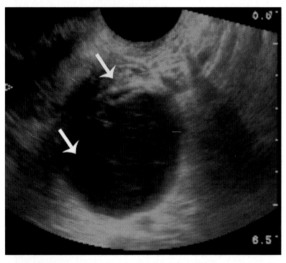

Hemorrhagic cyst: Hemorrhagic ovarian cyst (white arrow) with blood clot (yellow arrow). Note the reticular or weblike pattern within cyst, resulting from lysis of red blood cells.

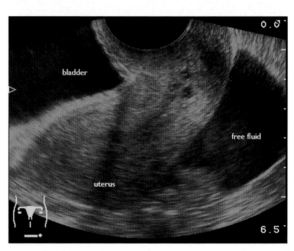

Hemorrhagic cyst: Transvaginal sonogram. Patient with ruptured hemorrhagic cyst with associated free fluid in the pelvic cul-de-sac (pouch of Douglas). Patients may present complaining of sudden onset of pelvic pain after intercourse.

Ovarian torsion

Ovarian torsion is the fifth most common gynecologic emergency. The risk of an adnexal mass to undergo torsion markedly increases at sizes > 4 cm. Absence or impaired ovarian venous flow on Doppler may be found in the setting of torsion.

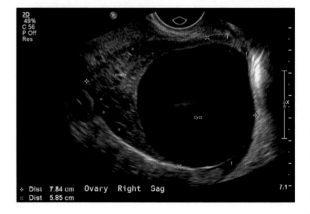

Ovarian torsion: Transvaginal sonogram. An 18-year-old female with intermittent right lower quadrant pain. Post-operative diagnosis of ovarian cyst and torsion. Right ovary with a 5.4 × 6.3 × 5.4 cm anechoic cyst. Note the enlarged ovary with multiple follicles (*) at the periphery and free fluid (f) surrounding the ovary.

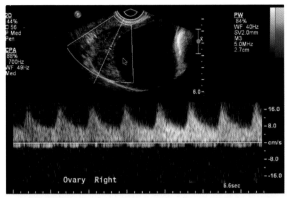

Ovarian torsion: Transvaginal sonogram. Sagittal view. An 18-year-old female with intermittent right lower quadrant pain. Post-operative diagnosis of ovarian cyst and torsion. Color Doppler can be used to evaluate ovarian arterial blood flow. Note the decreased blood flow to the ovary. However, approximately 50% of patients will have a normal Doppler flow study.

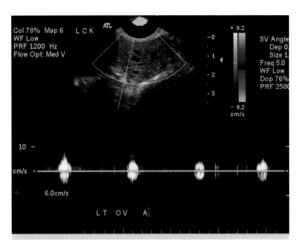

Ovarian torsion: Transvaginal sonogram. Ovarian torsion. Duplex ultrasound showing asymmetry of arterial waveforms with diminished diastolic component of the ovarian arterial flow.

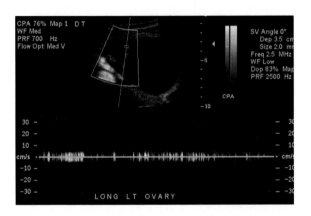

Ovarian torsion: A 12-year-old patient with ovarian torsion. Venous waveform measured. Note the decreased flow in the adnexal mass.

Fibroid uterus

Uterine leiomyomas are benign monoclonal tumors. They arise from the smooth cells of the myometrium. Fibroids are clinically relevant when they cause uterine enlargement greater than or equal to 9-weeks size, fibroid greater than or equal to 4 cm or submucosal fibroids. Transvaginal ultrasound has a high sensitivity (95–100%) for detecting fibroids. Fibroids appear heterogenous. When fibroids undergo necrosis, they may have anechoic components.

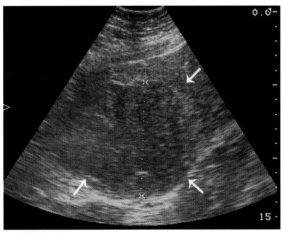

Fibroid uterus: Uterine leiomyoma.

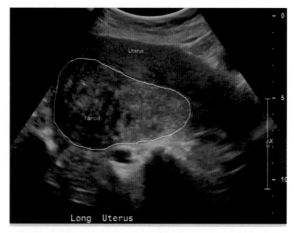

Fibroid uterus: Transabdominal sonogram. Longitudinal view. Uterine leiomyoma.

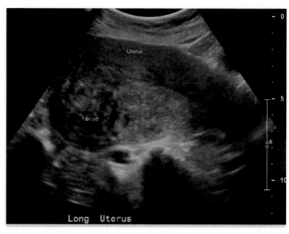

Fibroid uterus: Transabdominal sonogram. Longitudinal view. Uterine leiomyoma.

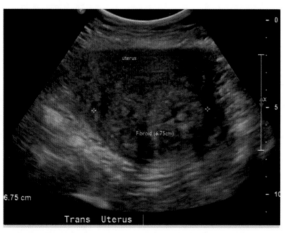

Fibroid uterus: Transabdominal sonogram. Transverse view. Uterine leiomyoma.

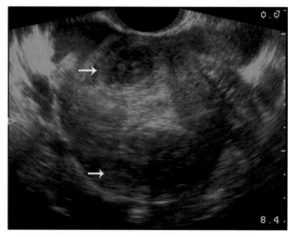

Fibroid uterus: Transverse sonogram. Multiple fibroids (arrows).

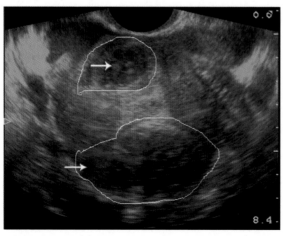

Fibroid uterus: Transverse sonogram. Multiple fibroids (arrows).

Genitourinary ultrasound

Christina Umber and John Christian Fox

Normal kidney

Renal ultrasound is an efficient way to screen the kidneys for major pathology. It is non-invasive and can be completed within minutes. Care must be taken to ensure that appropriate landmarks are found. The liver should be visualized adjacent to the right kidney and the spleen should be seen adjacent to the left kidney. Determination of normal renal anatomy can be accomplished through utilization of the renal border, pyramids, parenchyma and pelvis as markers.

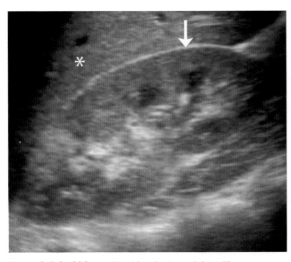

Normal right kidney: Renal border (arrow), liver (*).

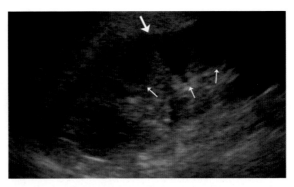

Normal renal pyramids: Renal pyramids (small arrows), renal border (large arrow).

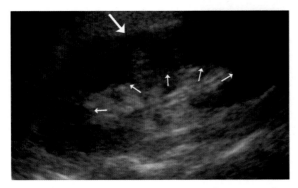

Normal renal pyramids: Renal pyramids (small arrows), renal border (large arrow).

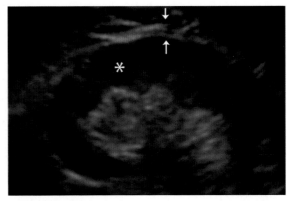

Perinephric fat: Perinephric fat (arrows), adipose capsule of the kidney, renal parenchyma (*).

Atlas of Emergency Ultrasound, ed. John Christian Fox. Published by Cambridge University Press. © J.C. Fox 2011.

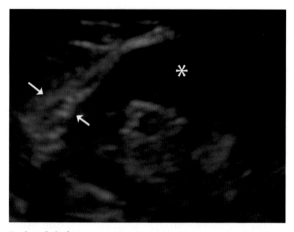

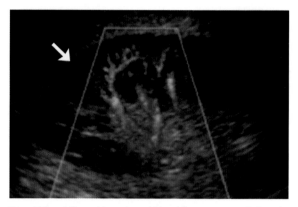

Perinephric fat: Perinephric fat (arrows), adipose capsule of the kidney, renal parenchyma (*).

Renal blood flow: Normal renal blood flow as seen with Doppler sonography (blue and red colors). Renal border (arrow).

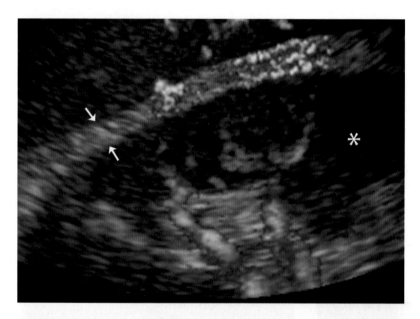

Renal blood flow: Renal blood flow as seen with Doppler sonography (blue and red colors). Renal parenchyma (*), perinephric adipose tissue (arrows).

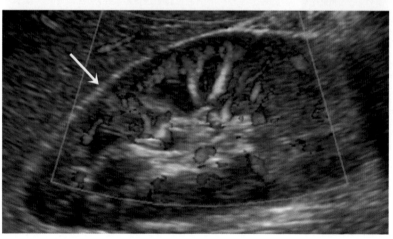

Renal blood flow: Normal blood flow of the kidney as seen with Doppler sonography (blue and red colors). Renal border indicated by arrow.

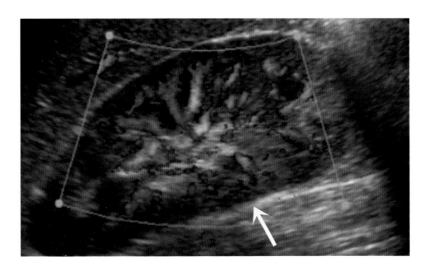

Renal blood flow: Normal blood flow of the kidney (blue and red colors). Renal border indicated by arrow.

Renal variation

Variation in the anatomical location and size of the kidneys as well as how they maintain vascularization does not necessarily predict pathology or symptoms. This is especially true when the anomaly is unilateral. Conversely, when symptoms are present, sonography is a quick way to screen for obvious anatomical pathology.

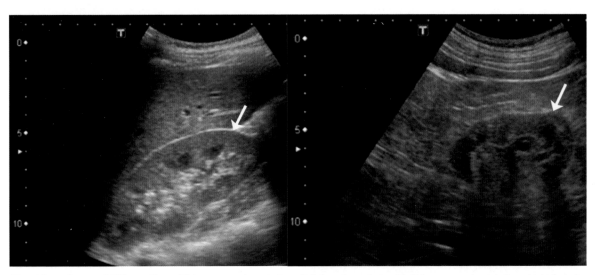

Atrophic and normal kidney: Normal kidney, approximately 5 cm (left frame); small atrophic kidney, approximately 3 cm (right frame). Renal borders indicated with arrows.

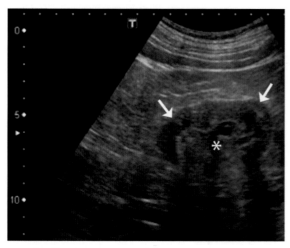

Atrophic kidney: Small atrophic kidney, approximately 3 cm, renal border (arrows), renal pelvis (*).

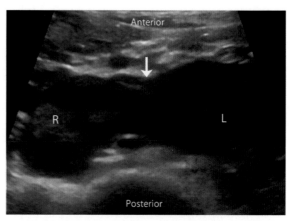

Horseshoe kidney: Right (R) and left (L) kidneys connected anterior to the spine by an isthmus (arrow) of renal tissue. This is a congenital anomaly that affects approximately 1 in 400 people.

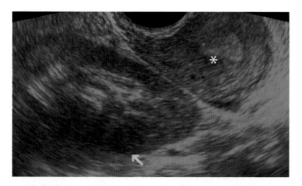

Pelvic kidney: Pelvic kidney (arrow) seen on endovaginal ultrasound. Uterus (*). It is estimated that in the United States 1 in every 500 births are affected by fetal pelvic kidney.

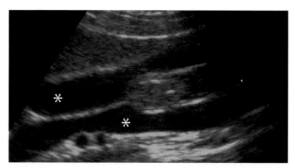

Duplicate renal arteries: Arterial lumens indicated by *. This anomaly is present in 15–20% of the general population.

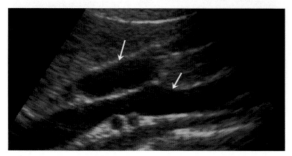

Duplicate renal arteries: Arterial borders indicated by arrows. This anomaly is present in 15–20% of the general population.

Renal masses, cysts, and abscesses

The kidneys may present with several forms of impinging anomalies. Differentiation between the various pathologies is initiated through ultrasound. The echogenicity of abnormal findings is the first step in determining the underlying pathology. A follow-up renal biopsy is frequently needed for definitive diagnosis.

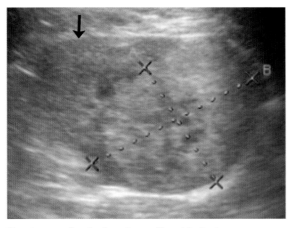

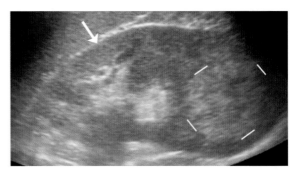

Renal mass: Renal cell carcinoma (between white lines; also known as hypernephroma) is a kidney cancer that originates in the lining of the proximal convoluted tubule. Renal border (arrow).

Renal mass: Renal cell carcinoma (A and B; also known as hypernephroma) is a kidney cancer that originates in the lining of the proximal convoluted tubule. Renal border (arrowhead).

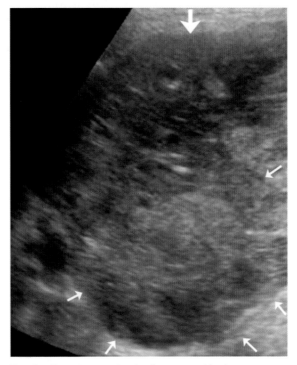

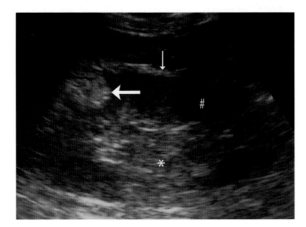

Renal mass: Renal cell carcinoma (large arrow) – (also known as hypernephroma) is a kidney cancer that originates in the lining of the proximal convoluted tubule. Renal border (small arrow). Parenchyma (#), pelvis (*).

Renal cell carcinoma: Renal cell carcinoma (also known as hypernephroma) is a kidney cancer that originates in the lining of the proximal convoluted tubule. Renal mass (small arrows), renal border (large arrow).

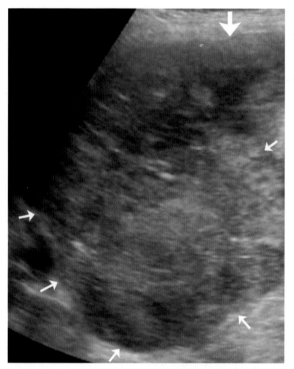

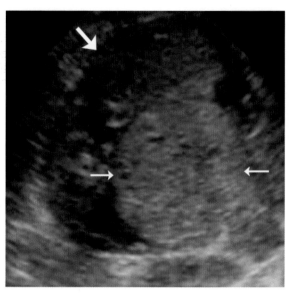

Wilms' tumor: Wilms' tumor (small arrows) or nephroblastoma is cancer of the kidneys that typically occurs in children, rarely in adults. Renal border (large arrow).

Renal cell carcinoma: Renal cell carcinoma (also known as hypernephroma) is a kidney cancer that originates in the lining of the proximal convoluted tubule. Renal mass (small arrows), renal border (large arrow).

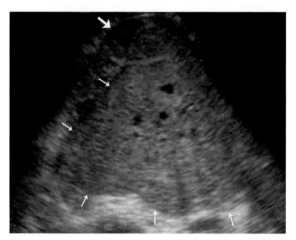

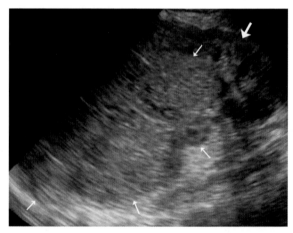

Wilms' tumor: Wilms' tumor (small arrows) or nephroblastoma is cancer of the kidneys that typically occurs in children, rarely in adults. Renal border (large arrow).

Wilms' tumor: Wilms' tumor (small arrows) or nephroblastoma is cancer of the kidneys that typically occurs in children, rarely in adults. Renal border (large arrow).

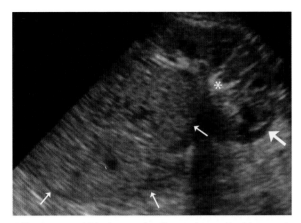

Wilms' tumor: Wilms' tumor (small arrows) or nephroblastoma is cancer of the kidneys that typically occurs in children, rarely in adults. Renal border (large arrow), renal pelvis (*).

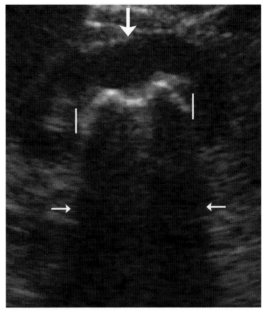

Renal calculus: Large renal calculus (between lines), acoustical shadowing (between small arrows), renal border (large arrow).

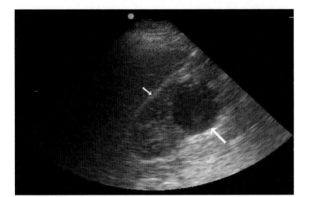

Renal cyst: Kidney (small arrow) with renal cyst (large arrow) – fluid collection in the kidney.

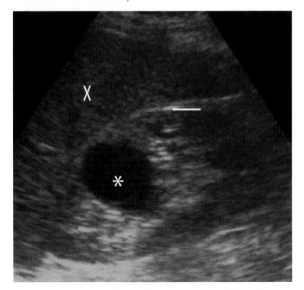

Renal cyst: Renal cyst (*) – fluid collection in the kidney. Renal border (white line), liver (X).

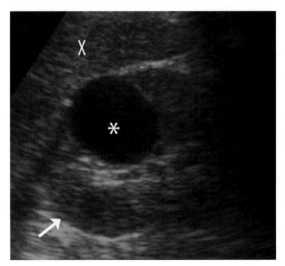

Renal cyst: Renal cyst (*) – fluid collection in the kidney. Renal border (arrow), liver (X).

109

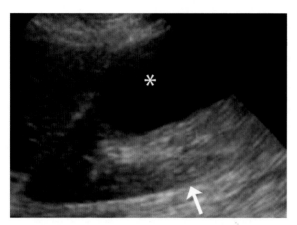

Renal cyst: Renal cyst (*) – fluid collection in the kidney. Renal border (arrow).

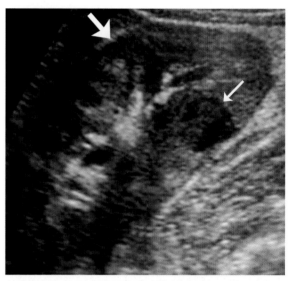

Renal abscess: Renal abscess (small arrow), renal border (large arrow).

Hydronephrosis and hydroureter

Hydronephrosis is distension and dilation of the renal pelvis and calyces, usually caused by obstruction of the free flow of urine from the kidney, leading to progressive atrophy of the kidney. Hydronephrosis can be seen as an enlarged area of decreased echogenicity usually originating at the renal pelvis and extending into the parenchyma.

Abnormal enlargement of the ureter by any blockage that prevents urine from draining into the bladder results in hydroureter. Normal ureter size is approximately 1.8 mm, when obstructed average width is 7 mm.

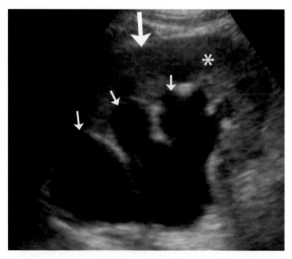

Moderate hydronephrosis: Dilated calyces (small arrows), renal parenchyma (*), renal border (large arrow).

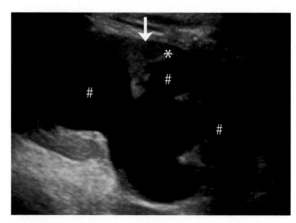

Severe hydronephrosis: Dilated calyces (#), compressed renal parenchyma (*), renal border (arrow).

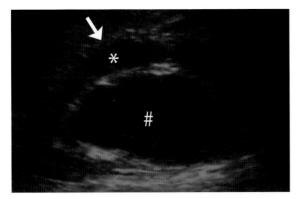

Severe hydronephrosis: Dilated calyx (#), compressed renal parenchyma (*), renal border (arrow).

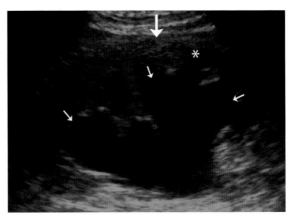

Massive hydronephrosis: Dilated renal calyces (small arrows), compressed renal parenchyma (*), renal border (large arrow).

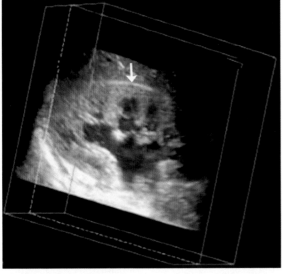

Hydronephrosis in 3D: Accumulation of urine in the kidney, as seen with 3-dimensional ultrasound. Renal border indicated by the arrow.

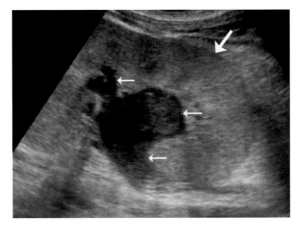

Hydronephrosis with debris: Accumulation of urine in the kidney with debris (fuzzy opacities) in the collecting system (small arrows). Renal border (large arrow).

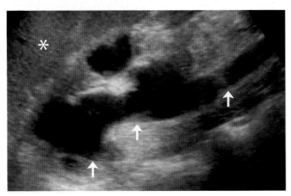

Hydronephrosis with debris: Accumulation of urine in the kidney with debris (fuzzy opacities) in the collecting system (arrows). Renal parenchyma (*).

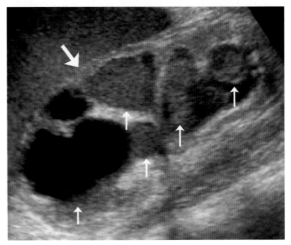

Hydronephrosis with debris: Accumulation of urine in the kidney with debris (fuzzy opacities) in the collecting system (small arrows). Renal border (large arrow).

111

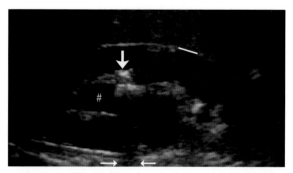

Hydronephrosis with stone: Hydronephrosis with renal calculus. Dilated calyx (#), calculus (large arrow), acoustic shadow (small arrows), renal border (white line).

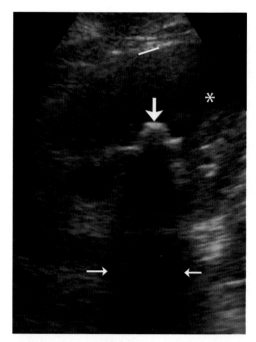

Hydronephrosis with stone: Hydronephrosis with renal calculus. Dilated calyx (*), calculus (large arrow), acoustic shadow (small arrows), renal border (white line).

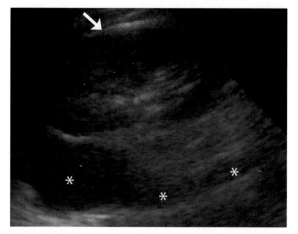

Hydroureter: Hydroureter without hydronephrosis. Dilated ureter (*), renal border (arrow).

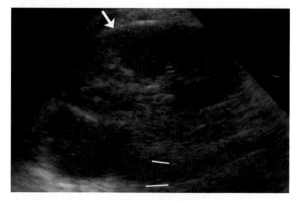

Hydroureter: Hydroureter without hydronephrosis. Dilated ureter (between white lines). Renal border (arrow).

Polycystic kidney disease

An inherited disorder that over time causes many grape-like clusters of fluid-filled cysts to form in both kidneys. Frequently patients have no symptoms and their physical condition appears normal for many years, so the disease can go unnoticed. Upon sonography it is seen as multiple cystic structures enveloping fluid seen as decreased echogenicity.

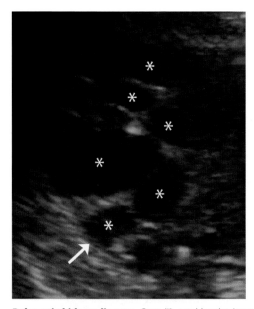

Polycystic kidney disease: Cysts (*), renal border (arrow).

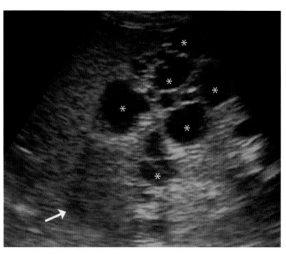

Polycystic kidney disease: Cysts (*), renal border (arrow).

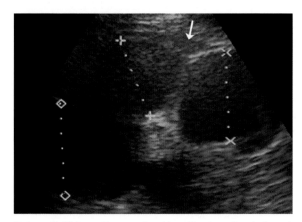

Polycystic kidney disease: Cysts (dotted lines), renal border (arrow).

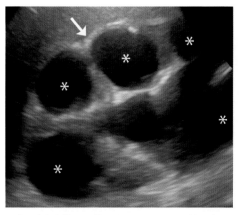

Polycystic kidney disease: Cysts (*), renal border (arrow).

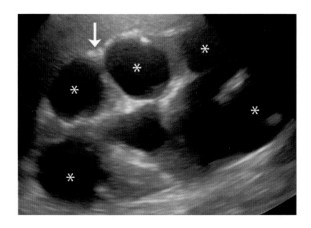

Polycystic kidney disease: Cysts (*), renal border (arrow).

Normal urinary bladder

Urinary bladder ultrasound is an efficient way to screen the bladder for major pathology. It is non-invasive and can be completed within minutes. The bladder is best visualized when full, with the probe immediately superior to the pubic symphysis angled inferiorly behind the pubic bone.

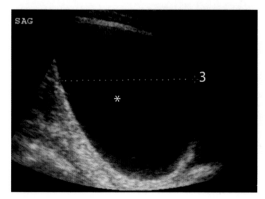

Bladder volume, sagittal plane: Urinary bladder volume measurement 3 is taken from the lumen of the bladder (*) in the sagittal plane. Measurements 1 and 2 are taken in the transverse plane.

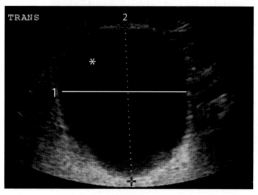

Bladder volume, transverse plane: Urinary bladder volume measurements 1 and 2 are taken from the lumen of the bladder (*) in the transverse plane. Measurement 3 is taken in the sagittal plane.

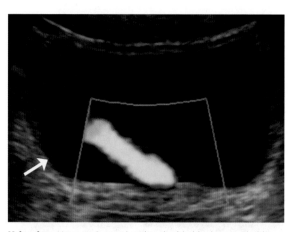

Urine jet: Urine jet (orange) within the bladder lumen. Bladder border (arrow).

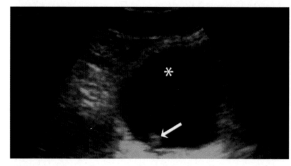

Urine jet: Over-gained urinary bladder (*) image demonstrating urine jet (arrow).

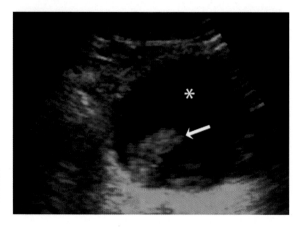

Urine jet: Over-gained urinary bladder (*) image demonstrating urine jet (arrow).

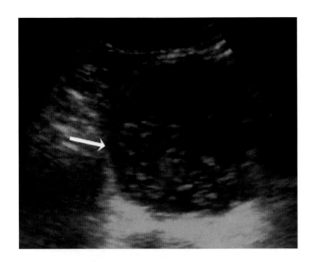

Urine jet: Over-gained urinary bladder (arrow) image demonstrating disbursement of urine jet (pale areas in the lumen of the bladder).

Urinary bladder variation

Various forms of disease pathology may affect the urinary bladder. Several major pathologies can be seen by ultrasound. Any increased echogenic areas within the bladder lumen may indicate the presence of a mass or calculi. Visualization of the bladder wall is also useful to screen for cystitis as well as impingement from the prostate.

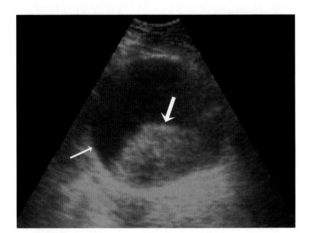

Bladder mass: Mass within the urinary bladder lumen (large arrow). Border of the bladder indicated by small arrow.

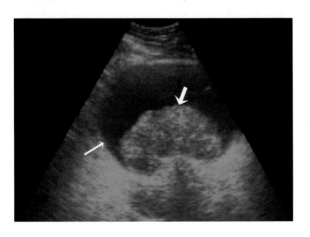

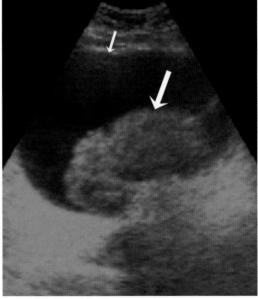

Bladder mass: Mass within the urinary bladder lumen (large arrow). Border of the bladder indicated by small arrow.

115

Bladder mass: Mass within the urinary bladder lumen (large arrow). Border of the bladder indicated by small arrow.

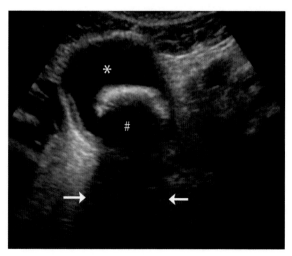

Bladder stone: Vesical calculus (bladder stone, #). Urinary bladder lumen (*). Acoustical shadow from stone (arrows).

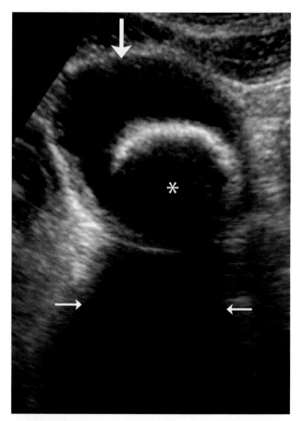

Bladder stone: Vesical calculus (bladder stone, *). Urinary bladder border (large arrow). Acoustical shadow from stone (small arrows).

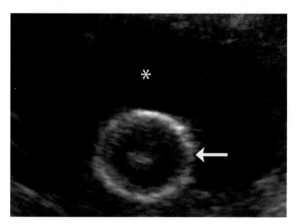

Foley catheter: Foley catheter (arrow) within the lumen of the urinary bladder (*).

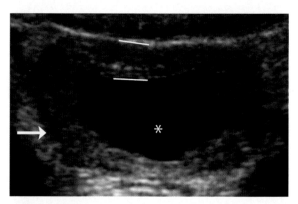

Pediatric cystitis: Inflammation of the urinary bladder. Thickened bladder wall (between lines). Urinary bladder lumen (*). Bladder border (arrow).

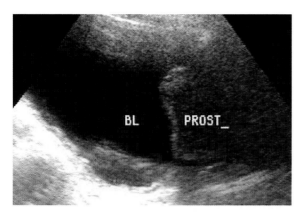

Enlarged prostate: Enlarged prostate (PROST) decreasing the volume of the urinary bladder lumen (BL). Normal prostate size is 4 × 2 × 3 cm.

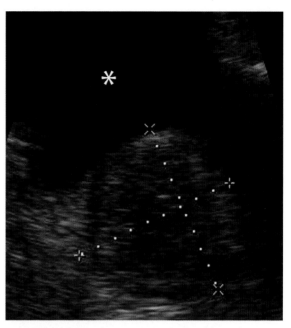

Enlarged prostate: Enlarged prostate (dotted lines). Urinary bladder lumen (*). Normal prostate size is 4 × 2 × 3 cm.

Normal testes

Testicular ultrasound is an efficient way to screen for major pathology. It is non-invasive and can be completed within minutes. It is frequently useful to visualize the asymptomatic testis as well as the affected testis when the patient presents with unilateral pathology. Initial visualization of both testes is accomplished utilizing a cleavage window.

Bilateral testes: Bilateral testes (*) in a single frame. Scrotum (#).

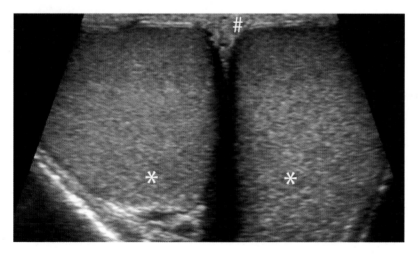

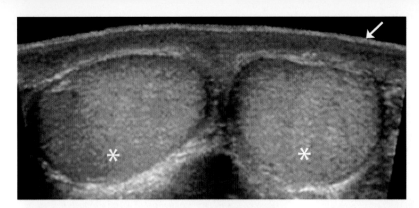

Bilateral testes: Bilateral testes (*) in a single frame. Scrotum (arrow).

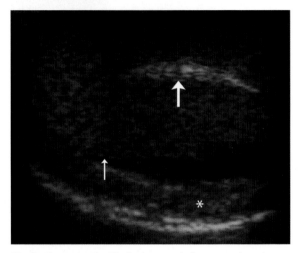

Mediastinum testis: Mediastinum testis (large arrow), testis border (small arrow), scrotum (*).

Mediastinum testis: Mediastinum testis (large arrow), testis border (small arrow), scrotum (*).

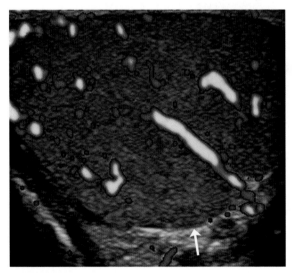

Testis blood flow: Normal testis blood flow (orange color), testis border (arrow).

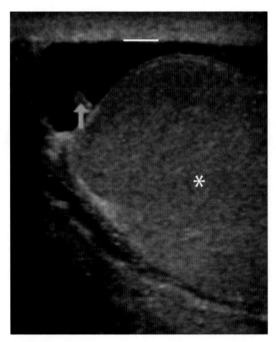

Appendix testis: Appendix testis (orange arrow), testis (*), scrotum border (white line). The appendix testis (or hydatid of Morgagni) is a vestigial remnant of the Müllerian duct, present on the upper pole of the testis and attached to the tunica vaginalis. It is present about 90% of the time.

Testes variation

There is a wide range of pathology that may affect the testes. Internal dilatations, internal and external trauma, hernias, and infections are a few of the disease processes that can be screened for with ultrasound.

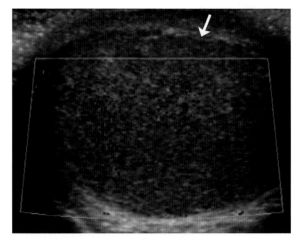

Testicular torsion: Orange coloring within the green lines indicates blood flow to the testis. A lack of blood flow is seen with testicular torsion. Testis border (arrow).

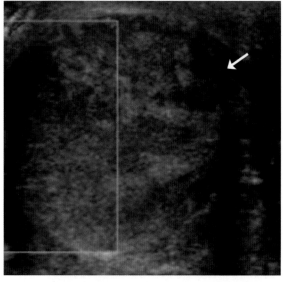

Torsion infarcted testis: Echoic variation throughout the testis caused by infarction secondary to torsion. Testis border (arrow).

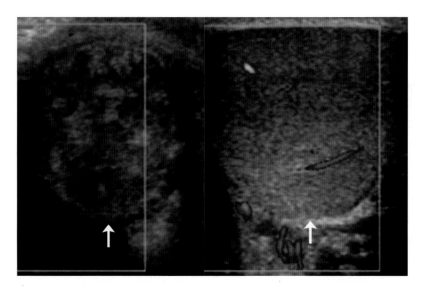

Torsion infarcted testis (left): Echoic variation throughout the testis caused by infarction secondary to torsion. Normal testis (right), testes borders (arrows).

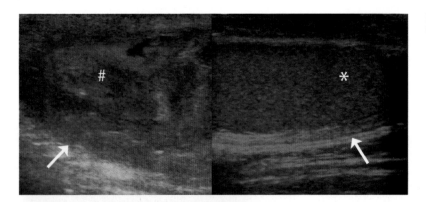

Fractured testis: Fractured testis (#), normal testis (*), testes borders (arrows).

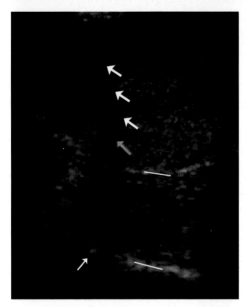

Gunshot wound to testis: Gunshot path (large arrows) with blood clot (between the white lines) within the scrotum (small arrow).

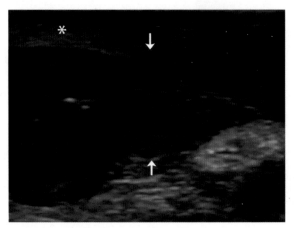

Scrotal hematoma: Scrotal hematoma (arrows), scrotum (*).

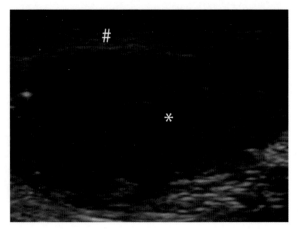

Scrotal hematoma: Scrotal hematoma (*), scrotum (#).

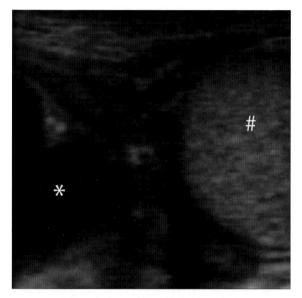

Inguinal hernia: The loop of bowel (*) is adjacent to the testis (#).

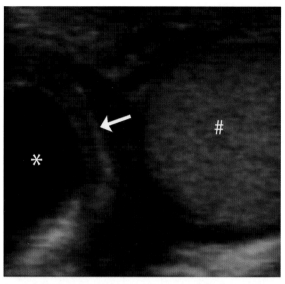

Inguinal hernia: The bowel wall (arrow) is adjacent to the testis (#). Bowel lumen (*).

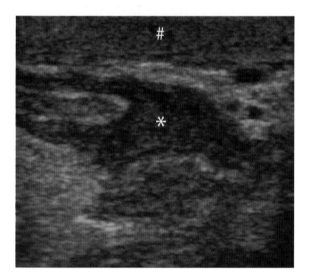

Scrotal hernia: Loop of bowel (*) in the scrotum (#). The testis is not in the frame.

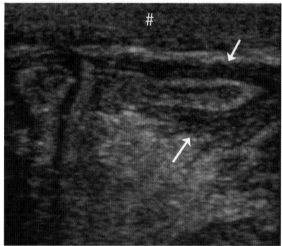

Scrotal hernia: Loop of bowel (arrows) in the scrotum (#). The testis is not in the frame.

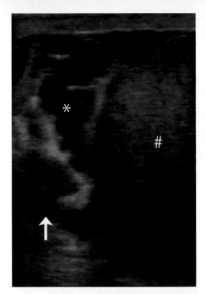

Spermatocele:
Retention cyst (*) in the head of the epididymis (arrow) distended with fluid that contains spermatozoa. Testis (#).

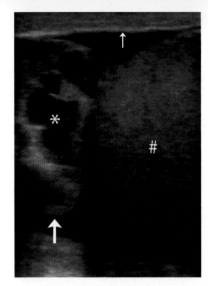

Spermatocele:
Retention cyst (*) in the head of the epididymis (large arrow) distended with fluid that contains spermatozoa. Testis (#), scrotum (small arrow).

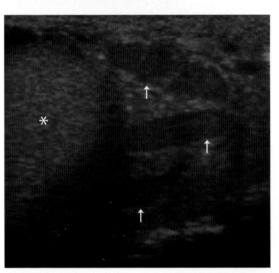

Varicocele: Dilatation of the veins associated with the spermatic cord in the testes. Dilated pampiniform plexus (arrows). Testis (*).

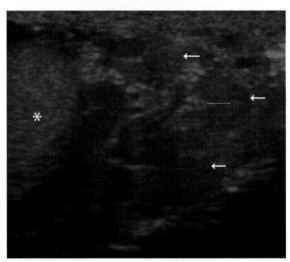

Varicocele: Dilatation of the veins associated with the spermatic cord in the testes. Dilated pampiniform plexus (arrows). Testis (*).

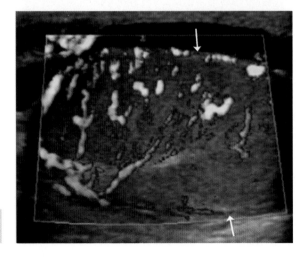

Orchitis: Increased blood flow (orange color) within the testis. Testis border (arrows).

Testicular masses, cysts, and abscesses

The testes may present with several forms of impinging anomalies. Differentiation between the various pathologies is initiated through ultrasound. The echogenicity of abnormal findings as well as their anatomical location are the first steps in determining the underlying pathology.

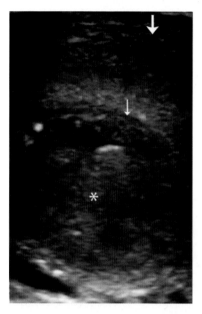

Testicular carcinoma: Testicular carcinoma (*), mass border (small arrow), testis border (large arrow).

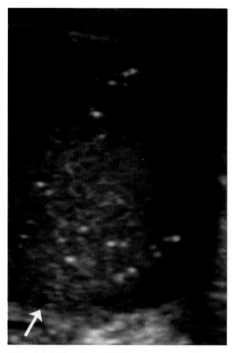

Microlithiasis: Microlithiasis is seen as small hyperechoic areas throughout the testis. Testis border (arrow). Testicular microlithiasis arises from microscopic calcium deposits within the testicles. It is not associated with risk of testicular cancer.

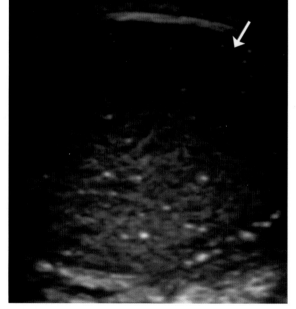

Microlithiasis: Microlithiasis is seen as small hyperechoic areas throughout the testis. Testis border (arrow). Testicular microlithiasis arises from microscopic calcium deposits within the testicles. It is not associated with risk of testicular cancer.

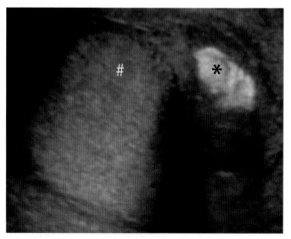

Extratesticular mass: Hyperechoic extratesticular mass (*) adjacent to normal testis (#).

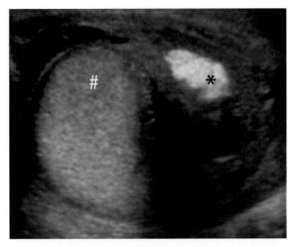

Extratesticular mass: Hyperechoic extratesticular mass (*) adjacent to normal testis (#).

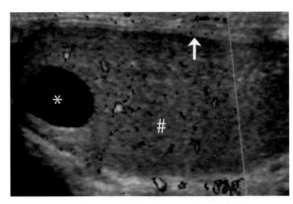

Intratesticular cyst: Intratesticular cyst (*), testis (#), scrotum (arrow).

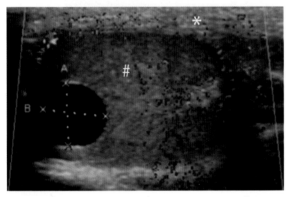

Intratesticular cyst: Intratesticular cyst (A & B), testis (#), scrotum (*).

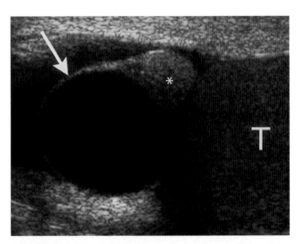

Epididymal cyst: Epididymal cyst (arrow), epididymis (*), testis (T).

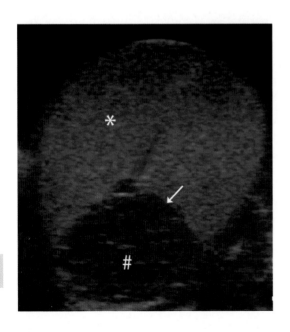

Tubular ectasia of rete testis: Benign tubular cysts (#), rete testis (arrow), testis (*).

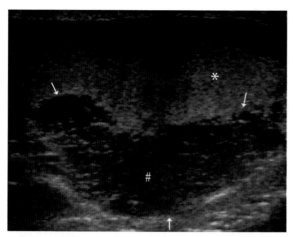

Tubular ectasia of rete testis: Benign tubular cysts (#), rete testis (arrows), testis (*).

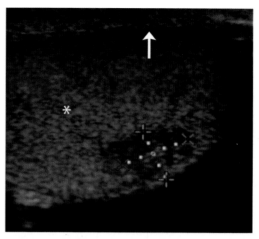

Testicular abscess: Testicular abscess (dotted lines), scrotum (arrow), testis (*).

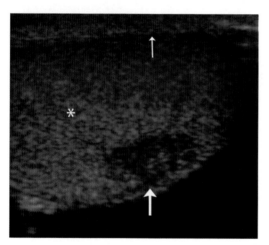

Testicular abscess: Testicular abscess (large arrow), scrotum (small arrow), testis (*).

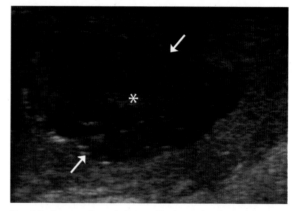

Scrotal abscess: Scrotal abscess (*), abscess border (arrows).

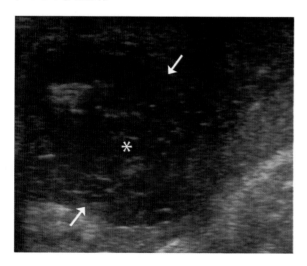

Scrotal abscess: Scrotal abscess (*), abscess border (arrows).

Hydrocele

A hydrocele is a fluid-filled sack along the spermatic cord within the scrotum. The main symptom is a painless, swollen testicle, which feels like a water balloon. It is seen on ultrasound as a region of decreased echogenicity surrounding the testis.

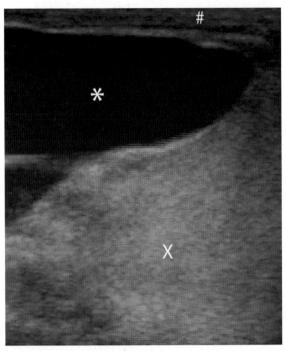

Hydrocele: Testis (X), scrotum (#), hydrocele fluid (*).

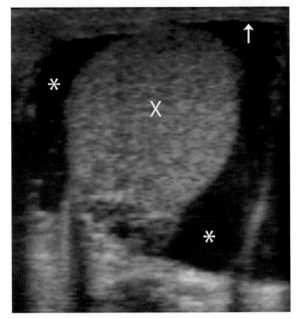

Hydrocele: Testis (X), scrotum (arrow), hydrocele fluid (*).

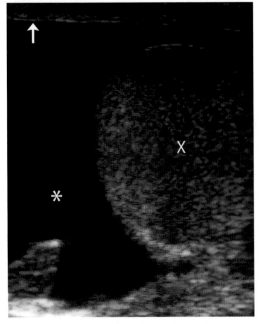

Hydrocele: Testis (X), scrotum (arrow), hydrocele fluid (*).

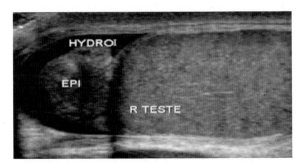

Hydrocele: Hydrocele (HYDRO), epididymis (EPI), right testis (R TESTE).

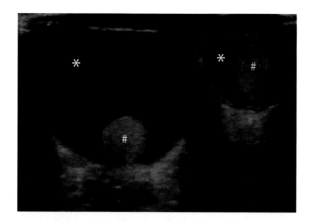

Bilateral hydroceles in an infant: Bilateral hydroceles (*) shown on cleavage window in 1-week-old with normal appearing testes (#).

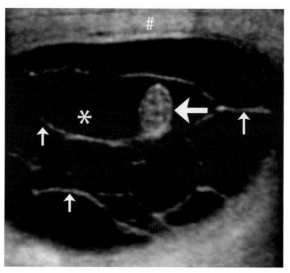

Loculated hydrocele: Epididymis (large arrow). Loculations, fibrous adhesions (small arrows), hydrocele fluid (*), scrotum (#).

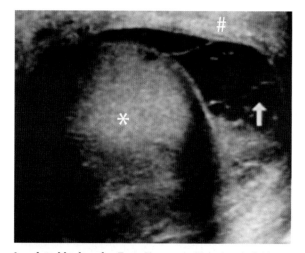

Loculated hydrocele: Testis (*), scrotum (#), hydrocele fluid (arrow) with loculations (thin gray lines), fibrous adhesions.

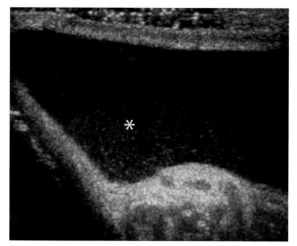

Hydrocele with debris: Hydrocele with debris (fuzzy appearing opacities) in the lumen (*).

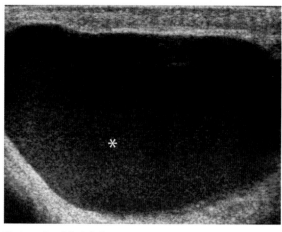

Hydrocele with debris: Hydrocele with debris (fuzzy appearing opacities) in the lumen (*).

Epididymitis

Epididymitis is inflammation of the epididymis, which stores and carries sperm. Pain and swelling are the most common signs and symptoms. Males of any age can get epididymitis, but it is most common in men between the ages of 20 and 39. In some cases, the testis may also become inflamed. This condition is called epididymo-orchitis. Upon sonography epididymitis presents as a thickened epididymis with increased blood flow.

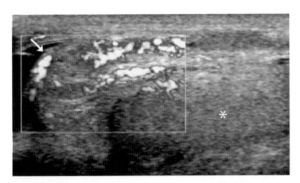

Epididymitis: Increased blood flow (orange color) in the epididymis (arrow). Testis (*).

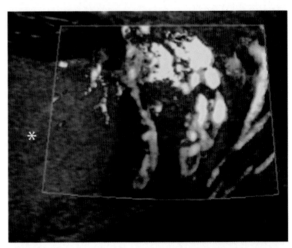

Epididymitis: Increased blood flow in the epididymis shown with orange color. Testis (*).

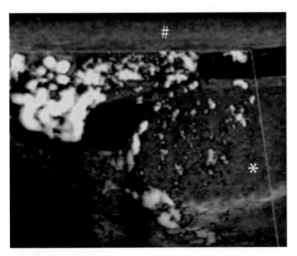

Epididymitis of head: Increased blood flow in the head of the epididymis shown with orange color. Testis (*), thickened scrotum (#).

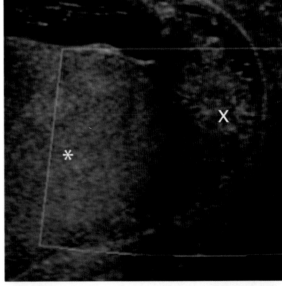

Epididymitis of tail: Thickened tail of the epididymis (X). Testis (*).

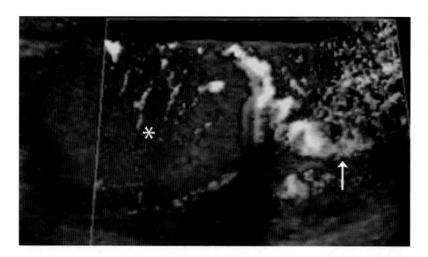

Epididymitis of tail: Increased blood flow in the tail of the epididymis (arrow) shown with orange color. Testis (*).

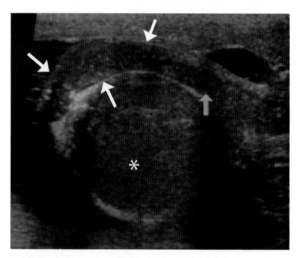

Epididymitis, coronal view: Thickened epididymis (arrows) adjacent to the testis (*).

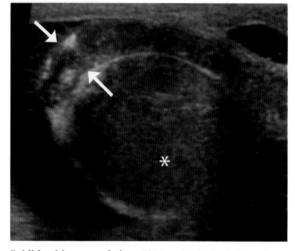

Epididymitis, coronal view: Thickened epididymis (between arrows) adjacent to the testis (*).

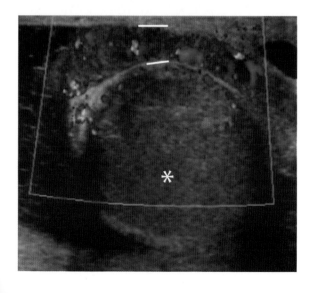

129

Epididymitis blood flow, coronal view: Blood flow through thickened epididymis (between white lines) adjacent to the testis (*).

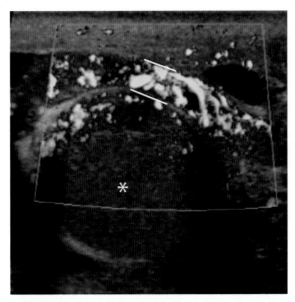

Epididymitis blood flow, coronal view: Increased blood flow (orange color) of epididymitis. Thickened epididymis (between white lines). Testis (*).

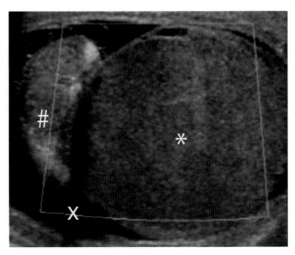

Epididymitis with hydrocele: Thickened epididymis (#). Hydrocele (X), a disorder in which serous fluid accumulates in a body sac (especially in the scrotum). Testis (*).

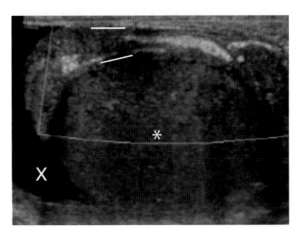

Epididymitis with hydrocele: Thickened epididymis (between white lines). Hydrocele (X), a disorder in which serous fluid accumulates in a body sac (especially in the scrotum). Testis (*).

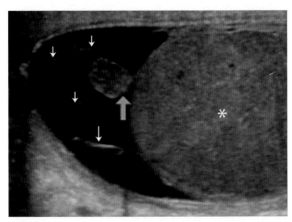

Epididymitis with loculated hydrocele: Thickened epididymis (large arrow). Loculation borders (small arrows), testis (*).

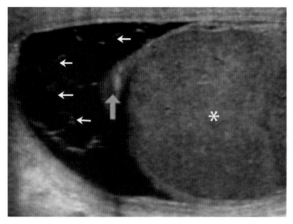

Epididymitis with loculated hydrocele: Thickened epididymis (large arrow). Loculation borders (small arrows), testis (*).

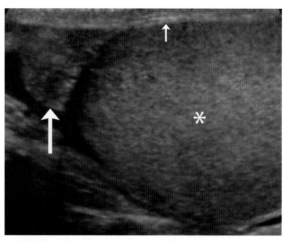

Epididymo-orchitis: Thickened epididymis (large arrow), enlarged testis (*), thickened scrotal skin (small arrow).

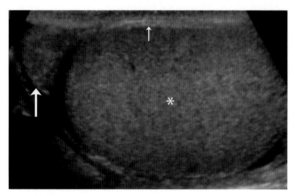

Epididymo-orchitis: Thickened epididymis (large arrow), enlarged testis (*), thickened scrotal skin (small arrow).

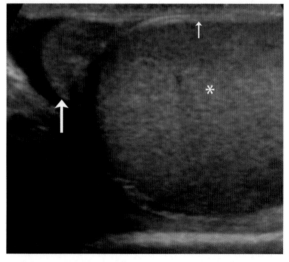

Epididymo-orchitis: Thickened epididymis (large arrow), enlarged testis (*), thickened scrotal skin (small arrow).

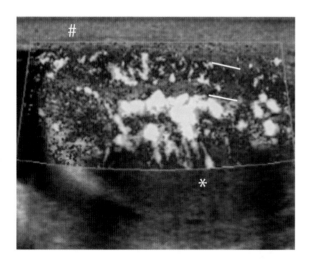

Epididymo-orchitis: Increased blood flow in both the epididymis and testis shown with orange color. Testis (*), thickened scrotum (#), epididymis (between white lines).

131

Penile fracture and penile implant

A penile fracture is an injury caused by the rupture of the tunica albuginea, which envelops the corpus cavernosum penis. It is most often caused by a blunt trauma to an erect penis. When ultrasound is performed rupture of the tunica albuginea and presence of a hematoma can be visualized.

Penile implants are seen as symmetric areas of increased echogenicity within the corpus cavernosum.

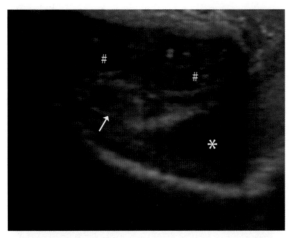

Penile fracture: Hematoma (*), corpus cavernosum (#), corpus spongiosum (arrow).

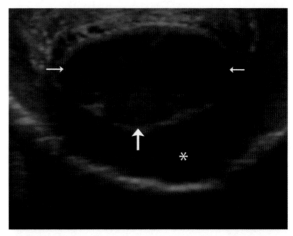

Penile fracture: Hematoma (*), corpus cavernosum (small arrows), corpus spongiosum (large arrow).

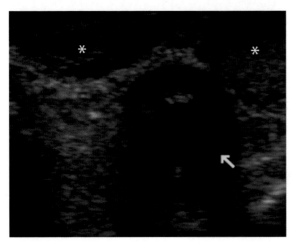

Penile implant: Penile implant (arrow), corpus cavernosum (*).

Musculoskeletal ultrasound

Deborah Shipley Kane and Jennifer McBride

Normal anatomy

Ultrasound can be used to view various bones, ligaments, tendons, and other musculoskeletal structures.

Here are several examples of normal anatomy. The normal anatomy can also be used for comparison with the abnormal extremity.

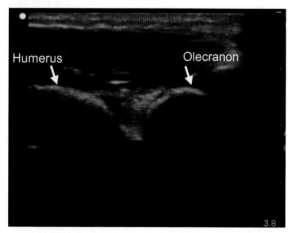

Normal shoulder: Compare the dislocated shoulder to this normal left anterior shoulder view. Here the proximal humerus is seen close to, and well aligned with, the glenoid fossa.

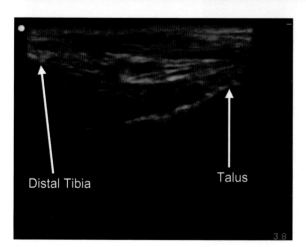

Normal ankle: Long axis of anterior ankle without effusion. Arrows pointing toward the tibia and the talus.

Normal elbow: Long axis of posterior elbow. Here one can see the smooth lines of the distal humerus and the olecranon (arrows).

Atlas of Emergency Ultrasound, ed. John Christian Fox. Published by Cambridge University Press. © J.C. Fox 2011.

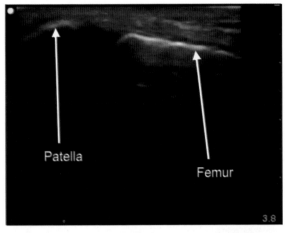

Normal knee: Long axis of anterior knee. Both the distal femur and the patella are seen in this image (arrows).

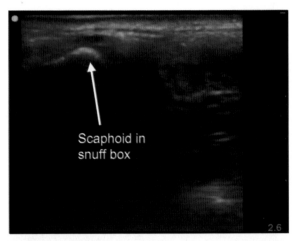

Normal scaphoid: This image of the scaphoid was taken with the probe in the anatomical snuffbox. Notice the normal hyperechoic scaphoid.

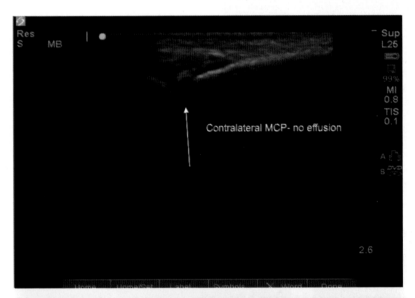

Normal MCP joint: Here is the contralateral right metacarpophalangeal joint without effusion. No dark/anechoic fluid is seen in this joint.

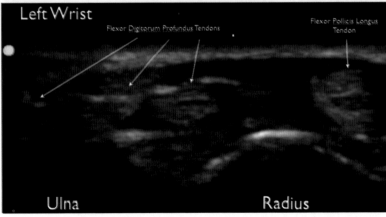

Wrist anatomy: Transverse/short axis of distal left wrist. Notice the short axis of multiple tendons as well as the radius and ulna.

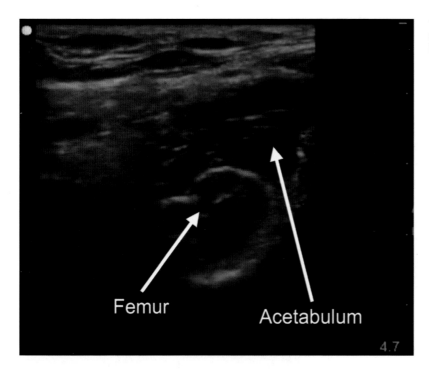

Transverse hip: Transverse view of anterior hip. Here the femur can be seen lying within the acetabulum.

Fractures and dislocations

Bone is easily visualized by ultrasound, and appears bright/hyperechoic. Fractures look like an incontinuity of the normally smooth line. Dislocations are noted when the bone/joint are not in normal alignment.

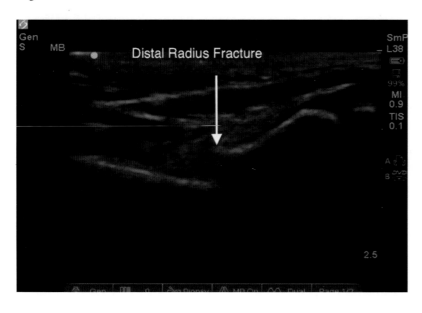

Distal radius fracture: Long axis. The bone appears as a hyperechoic line. The discontinuity of this line represents the fracture line seen above.

135

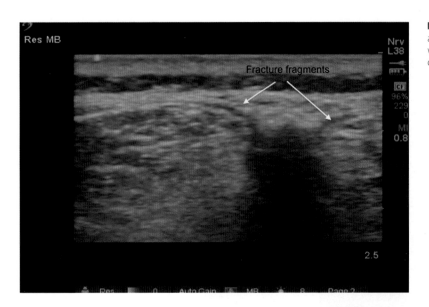

Femur fracture: Long axis. Proximal and distal fracture fragments are visible with large fracture line, representing displacement.

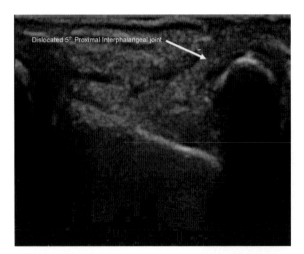

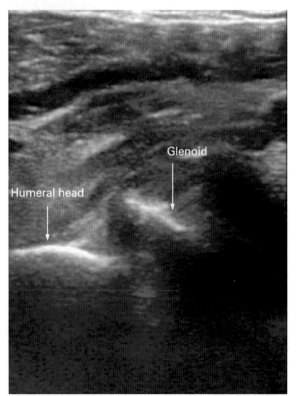

Dislocated finger: Notice the long, straight, hyperechoic (bright white) line in this picture, which is the proximal phalanx of the fifth digit. Then notice the arrow pointing toward the dislocated proximal interphalangeal joint. Normally these two bones would be aligned.

Shoulder dislocation: This is an image of the anterior right shoulder of a patient with an anterior shoulder dislocation. The proximal rounded humeral head is readily seen; although notice the separation from the glenoid fossa representing dislocation. Compare this to the contralateral normal left shoulder.

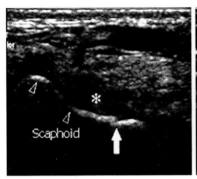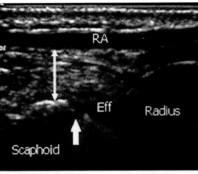

Scaphoid fracture: Left: Long axis of the scaphoid. Bold arrow represents the fracture line. Also a small effusion is seen around bone. Right: Short axis of the scaphoid, again the bold arrow is pointing toward the fracture line. Effusion (Eff), radial artery (RA).

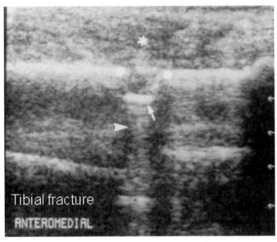

Tibial fracture: Fracture line is depicted with arrows. Notice a displacement of the fracture fragment.

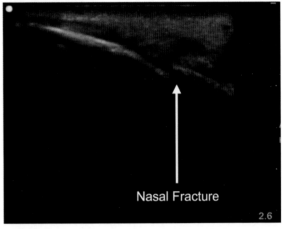

Nasal fracture: Sagittal/long axis view of the anterior nose. The arrow, representing a non-displaced nasal fracture, shows a break in the hyperechoic line of bone.

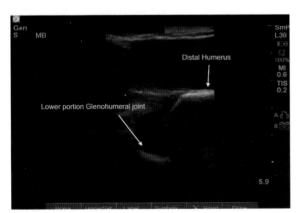

Dislocated shoulder: Another image of a dislocated right shoulder. Here the separation of the distal humerus with the shoulder joint is readily noticeable. Only the lower portion of the glenohumeral joint is seen in this image.

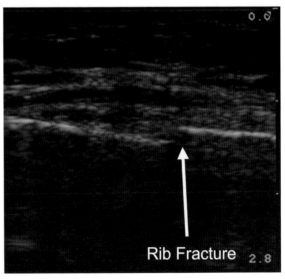

Rib fracture: Anterior right rib fracture. The ultrasound probe was placed over the tender area – fracture line represented by arrow.

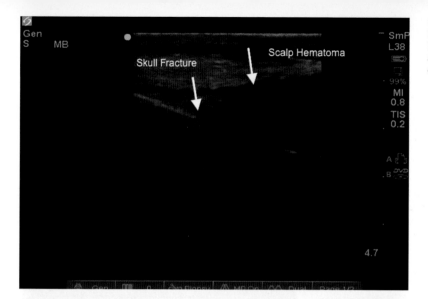

Skull fracture: Image of posterior skull in trauma patient with skull fracture. The beginning of the fracture line is noted by arrow, but is slightly distorted by large overlying scalp hematoma.

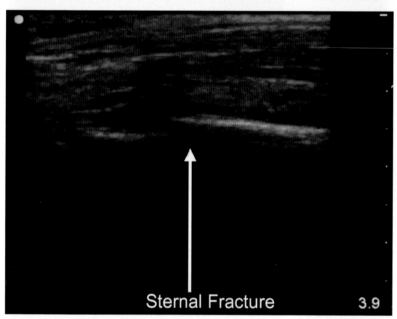

Sternal fracture: Long axis of anterior sternum. Arrow points to the fracture line.

Joint and ligament pathology

Ultrasound can also be utilized to visualize other pathology; including effusions, tendon/ligament ruptures, and foreign bodies. Fluid appears anechoic/black on ultrasound. Tendons and ligaments appear as a bundle of alternating hypo- and hyperechoic lines. In addition, foreign bodies can often be seen under ultrasound. If the structure is very small and superficial, a waterbath may be helpful.

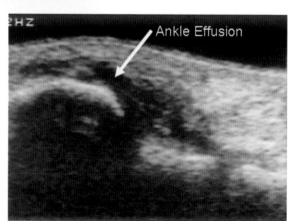

Ankle effusion: Hyperechoic bone is surrounded by anechoic fluid representing an effusion. This is an image of the long axis of the distal tibia.

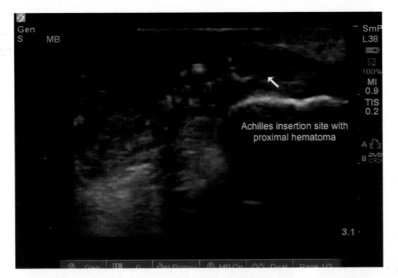

Ruptured Achilles tendon: Still image of a ruptured Achilles tendon. Long axis of posterior ankle. Achilles tendon seen proximal to bone (arrow); and appears as linear hypoechoic structure. Notice the abrupt end of this structure, representing the rupture. A small hematoma is noted by the rupture.

Achilles insertion site with proximal hematoma

3.1

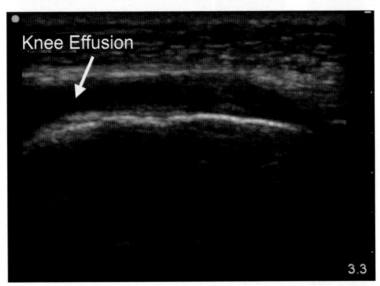

Knee effusion: Sagittal/long axis view of the proximal, anterior knee. An effusion is seen anterior to the hyperechoic bone.

Knee Effusion

3.3

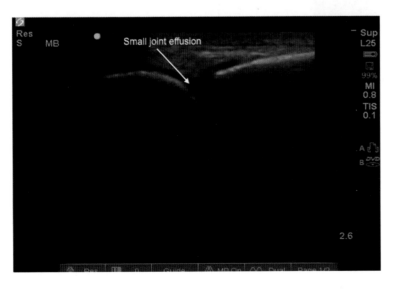

Gout: Left metacarpophalangeal joint in a patient diagnosed with gout. The arrow is pointing to a small joint effusion. Also notice some dark fluid within the surrounding tissue, possibly representing inflammation. This may be more noticeable when compared to the contralateral side.

Small joint effusion

2.6

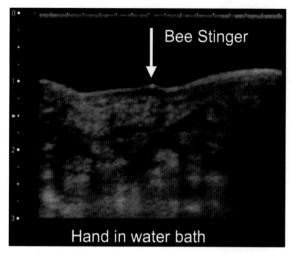

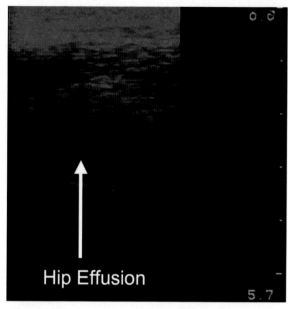

Hand in water bath: This technique is used to increase the resolution of small, superficial structures. Here a finger is placed under water, and the ultrasound probe is placed shallower in the water bath – to allow the water to be used as a sonographic window. Now, one can notice the hyperechoic superficial structure under the skin, which is a bee stinger in this patient.

Hip effusion: This is a transverse view of the anterior hip. The effusion is seen anterior to the bone as dark fluid.

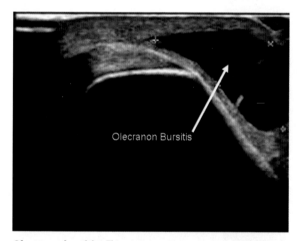

Olecranon bursitis: This picture represents an image of the posterior elbow in long axis. The bursa (arrow) is filled with anechoic (dark) material, which is fluid.

Pediatric ultrasound

Stephanie Doniger and George Mittendorf

Appendicitis

Ultrasound can be used as a method to diagnose acute appendicitis without placing the patient at the risk of radiation. The appendix can be seen as a blind ended tubular structure. With acute appendicitis, the inflamed appendix is noncompressible, has an increased diameter, and often contains an appendicolith.

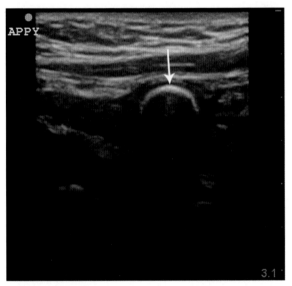

Acute appendicitis: Acute appendicitis with large appendicolith (arrow).

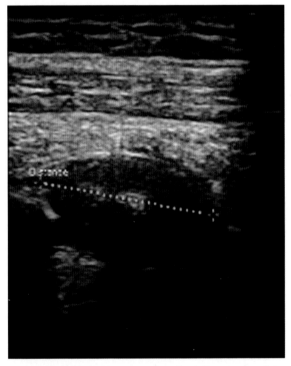

Acute appendicitis: Transverse view of an inflamed appendix in acute appendicitis.

Atlas of Emergency Ultrasound, ed. John Christian Fox. Published by Cambridge University Press. © J.C. Fox 2011.

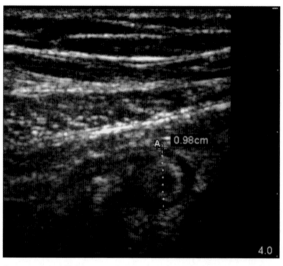

Acute appendicitis: Incompressible appendix without perforation.

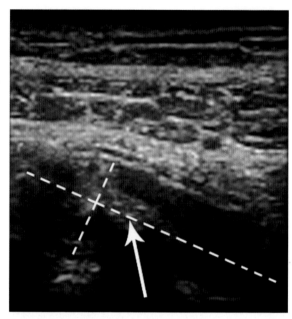

Acute inflammation: Longitudinal view of acute inflammation of appendix (long line). Diameter of appendix (short line). Fecalith (arrow).

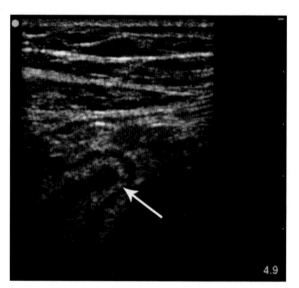

Acute appendicitis: The blind-ended, noncompressible tubular structure is consistent with acute appendicitis.

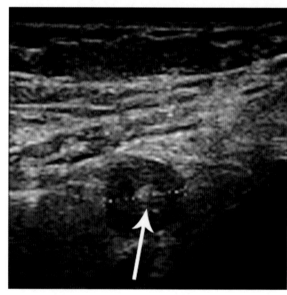

Acute appendicitis: Transverse view of acute appendicitis with central fecalith (arrow): Diameter is greater than 6 mm (dotted line).

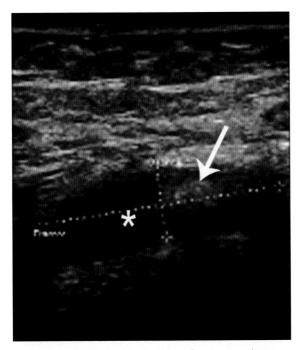

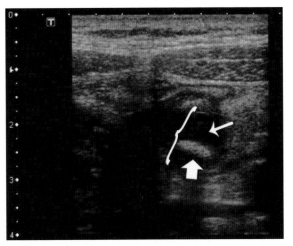

Acute appendicitis: Acute appendicitis in a 15-year-old male. Appendiceal lumen (skinny arrow), fecalith (fat arrow), diameter ("{").

Acute appendicitis: Longitudinal view of acute appendicitis. Fluid filled tubular appendix (asterisk), fecalith (arrow).

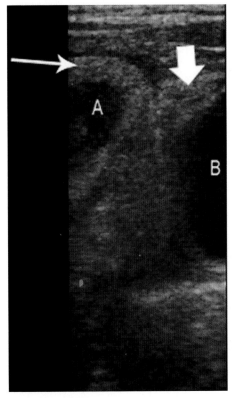

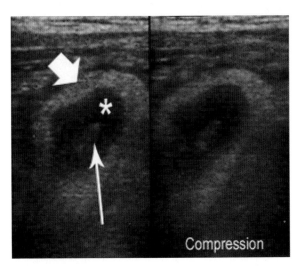

Acute appendicitis: Longitudinal view of acute appendicitis. Fluid filled lumen (asterisk). Fecalith (skinny arrow), inflamed appendiceal wall (fat arrow). The left panel shows the appendix prior to graded compression, while the right panel is after graded compression. Note that the appendix does not compress.

Acute appendicitis: Inflamed appendix adjacent to bladder. Lumen of appendix (A), lumen of bladder (B), inflamed appendiceal wall (skinny arrow), inflamed bladder wall (fat arrow).

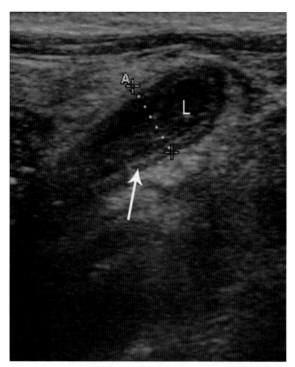

Child with acute appendicitis: Diameter of appendix = 1.03 cm (A). Lumen (L), appendiceal wall (arrow).

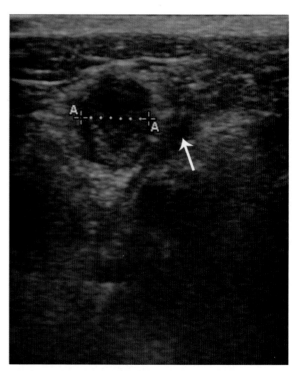

Child with acute appendicitis: Transverse view. Diameter of appendix is 0.92 cm (A). Free fluid (arrow).

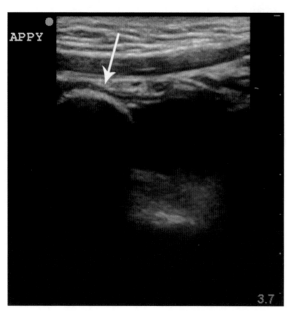

Acute appendicitis: Longitudinal view of a largely inflamed appendix with appendicolith.

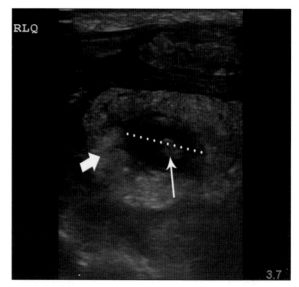

Acute appendicitis: Transverse view of perforated acute appendicitis. Appendiceal diameter, lumen of appendix (skinny arrow), surrounding abscess (fat arrow).

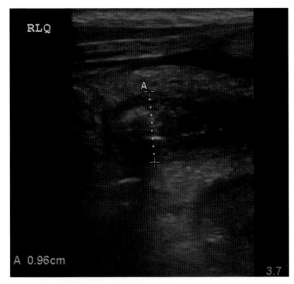

Acute appendicitis: Longitudinal view.

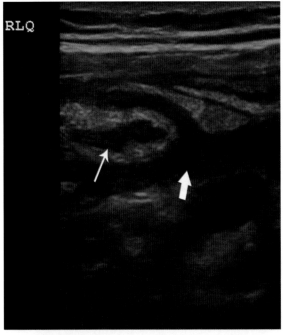

Acute appendicitis with perforation: Appendix (skinny arrow), surrounding abscess (fat arrow).

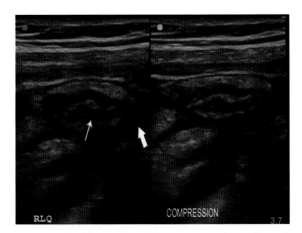

Acute appendicitis with perforation: Appendix (small arrow) with surrounding abscess (large arrow). Image on right is with compression.

Acute appendicitis with perforation: Inflamed appendiceal wall (skinny arrow), appendiceal lumen (asterisk), surrounding abscess (fat arrow).

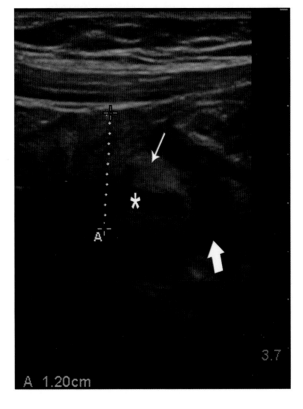

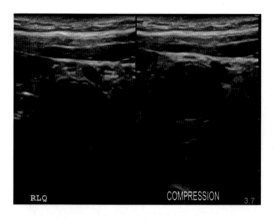

Acute appendicitis: Transverse view of an acutely inflamed appendix. The left panel demonstrates the appendix before graded compression, and the right panel is after graded compression. Note that the appendix does not compress.

Infection

Ultrasound can be used to evaluate various types of infections in pediatric patients. Skin infections can be studied to distinguish cellulitis from abscesses, which will aid in patient management.

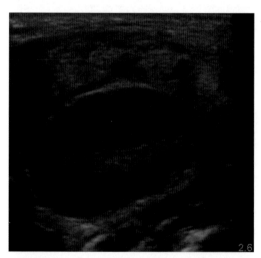

Child with cervical lymphadenitis: Enlarged lymph node demonstrating a hyperechoic center.

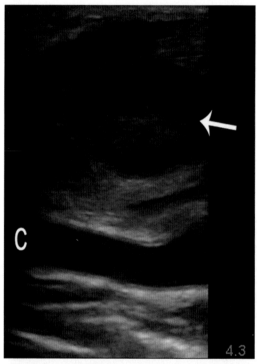

Cervical lymphadenitis: Cervical lymphadenitis (arrow) in close proximity to carotid artery (C).

Cellulitis

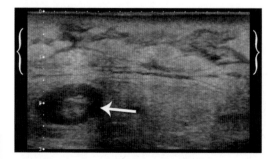

Cellulitis: Cellulitis ("{}"), lymph node (arrow).

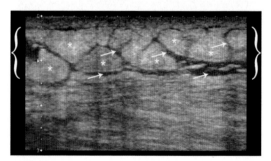

Cellulitis: Cellulitis in right calf with "cobblestoning" ("{}"). Hyperechoic subcutaneous tissue (asterisks) with subcutaneous edema filling the interlobar septae (arrows).

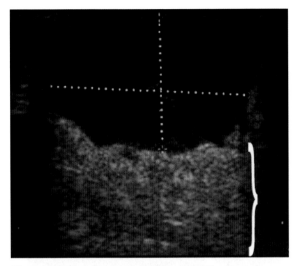

Abscess: Abscess on buttock (dotted cross) with expected increased echogenicity deep to the lesion ("}").

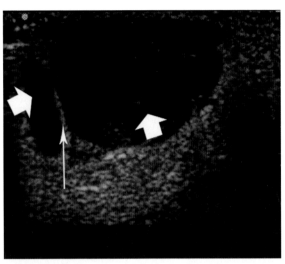

Abscess: A 2 cm × 3 cm abscess on buttock. Loculated abscess (fat arrows) with septations (skinny arrow).

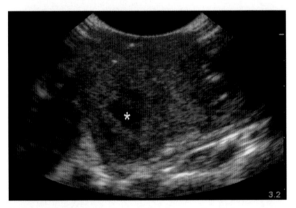

Peritonsillar abscess: Peritonsillar abscess after drainage with 18-gauge needle. Residual lumen (asterisk).

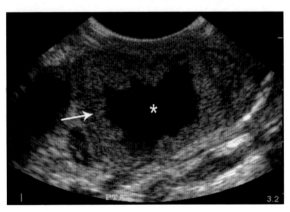

Peritonsillar abscess: A 17-year-old female with a peritonsillar abscess. Hypoechoic debris within abscess (asterisk), abscess capsule (arrow).

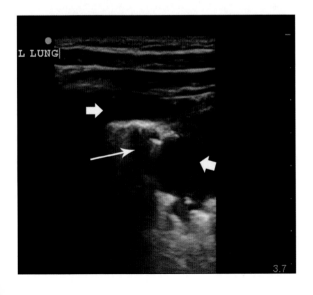

Pneumonia: Girl with pneumonia, loculated pleural effusions (fat arrows), and bright echoes with posterior acoustic shadowing consistent with air bronchograms (skinny arrow).

147

Intussusception

Intussusception can be viewed by ultrasound as a swirling mass of telescoping bowel. Alternating hyperechoic and hypoechoic layers represent the intussuscipiens and the intussusceptum. Both transverse and longitudinal views are valuable in demonstrating this morphology.

Infant with intussusception: Classic "target sign" with hyperechoic ileum (skinny arrow) telescoping into the outer hyperechoic ascending colon (fat arrow). Lumen of colon with fecal matter (small arrows).

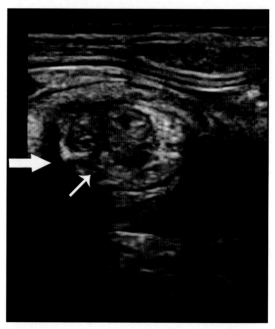

Infant with intussusception: Transverse view of right upper quadrant. Hyperechoic small bowel in center (small arrow) surrounded by a layer of hypoechoic cecal lumen (large arrow).

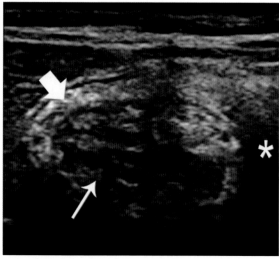

Infant with intussusception: Small bowel (small arrow) telescoping into the cecum (large arrow) with surrounding hypoechoic colic fluid (asterisk).

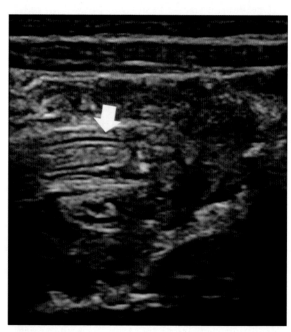

Child with intussusception: Longitudinal view of intussusceptum.

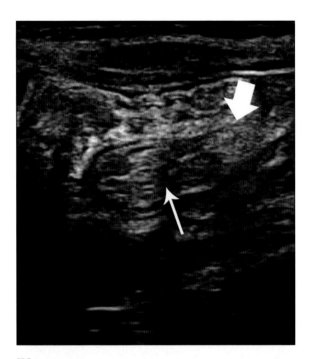

Intussusception: Longitudinal view. Pseudokidney (small arrow), start of intussusceptum (large arrow).

IV access

Obtaining intravenous access in the pediatric patient is often a difficult task. Ultrasound can be a valuable tool in this procedure.

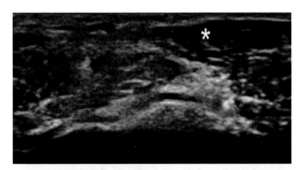

Brachial vein: Brachial vein after compression (asterisk).

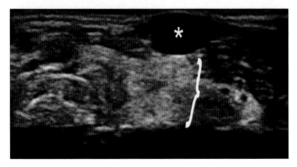

Brachial vein: Brachial vein before compression (asterisk) with posterior acoustic enhancement ("}").

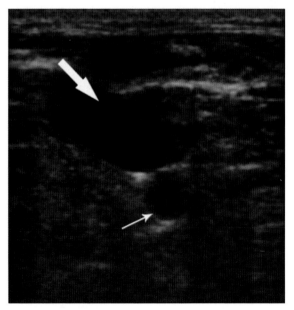

Internal jugular vein: Internal jugular vein with tenting during needle entry (large arrow), common carotid artery (small arrow).

Miscellaneous

The following section includes various implementations of ultrasound including cardiac, foreign bodies, and genitourinary applications.

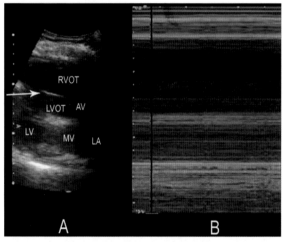

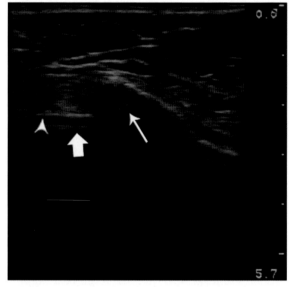

Asystole during a FAST scan of a trauma patient: (A) Left parasternal long axis view. Right ventricular outflow tract (RVOT), left ventricle (LV), septum (arrow), left ventricular outflow tract (LVOT), aortic valve (AV), mitral valve (MV), left atrium (LA). (B) Motion mode displaying cardiac standstill.

BB: BB implanted near heart (skinny arrow). Parietal pericardium (arrowhead). Epicardium (fat arrow).

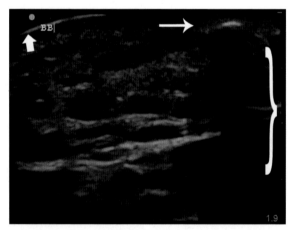

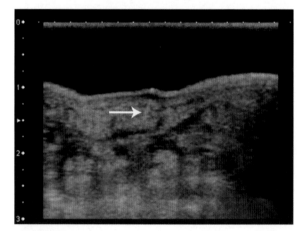

BB: BB (arrow) lodged just beneath the skin (fat arrow) with posterior acoustic shadowing (bracket).

Bee stinger: Bee stinger (arrow) seen in water bath.

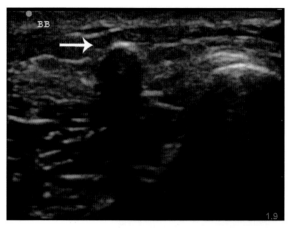

BB: BB lodged within soft tissue with posterior acoustic shadowing.

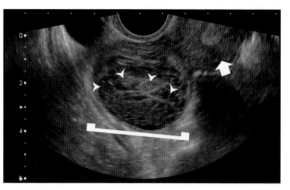

Ovarian mass: Transvaginal view of ovarian mass with individualized locules (arrowheads). Ovary ("{"), uterus (fat arrow).

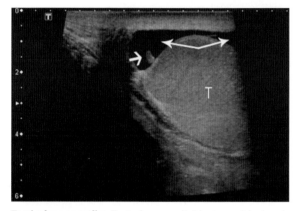

Testicular appendix: Testicular appendix (short arrow), hydrocele (double arrow), testicle (T).

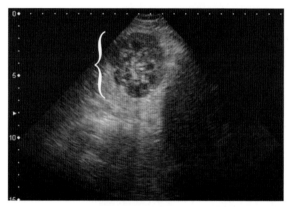

Wilms' tumor: Inferior aspect of Wilms' tumor ("{") in a 3-year-old patient.

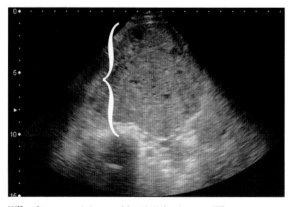

Wilms' tumor: A 3-year-old with Wilms' tumor ("{").

Pyloric stenosis

Pyloric stenosis usually presents at roughly 3 weeks after birth with nonbilious projectile vomiting. It is recommended that any infant with these symptoms have ultrasound evaluation immediately because the sensitivity and specificity for this diagnostic tool is close to 100%. Transverse and longitudinal views will demonstrate hypertrophied muscle and a narrow pyloric channel.

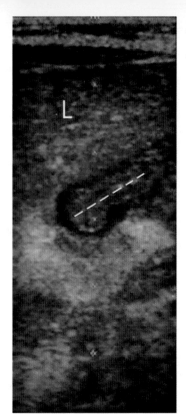

Pylorus: Longitudinal view of pylorus in healthy infant, pyloric canal lumen (dotted line), liver (L).

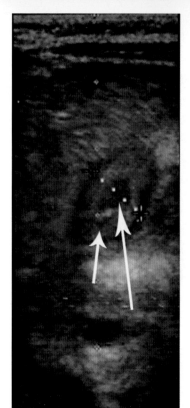

Normal pylorus: Cross-section of normal pylorus in healthy infant. Pylorus (short arrow), gastric lumen (long arrow).

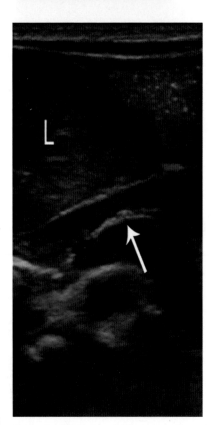

Normal pylorus: Longitudinal view of normal pylorus. Gastric contents are traversing the pyloric canal (arrow). Liver (L).

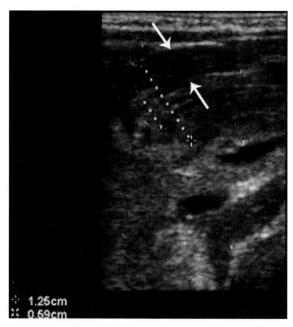

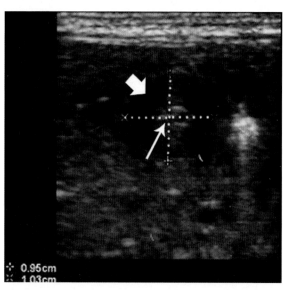

Pyloric stenosis: Infant with pyloric stenosis, cross-sectional view. Diameter of pylorus, lumen of pyloric canal (arrow), hypertrophied pyloric muscle (fat arrow).

Pyloric stenosis: Infant with pyloric stenosis. Duodenal width (shorter line), hypertrophic pylorus muscle (longer line), wall thickness of pylorus (between arrows).

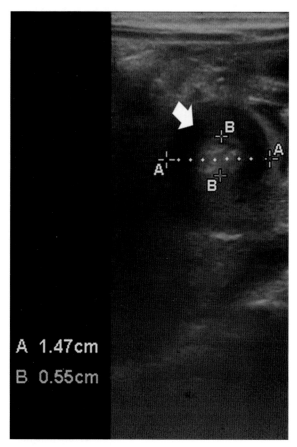

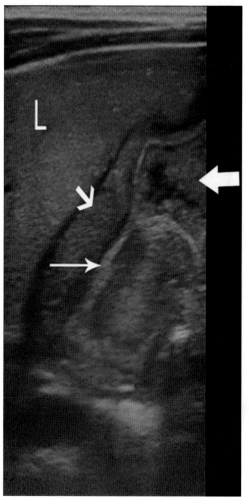

Pyloric stenosis: Diameter of pylorus (A) and pyloric canal (B). Hypertrophied pyloric muscle (arrow).

Pyloric stenosis: Hypertrophied pyloric muscle (short arrow), pyloric canal (skinny arrow), gastric lumen (fat arrow), liver (L).

Trauma

Ultrasound has become an important part of evaluating the trauma patient. In addition to detecting free fluid with the FAST scan, ultrasound can also be used to detect fractures. Furthermore, Doppler can be applied to quickly assess vascular function at the site of the injury.

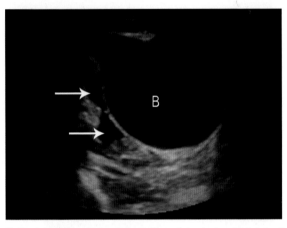

Patient with handlebar injury: Transabdominal sagittal view of bladder (B) with surrounding free fluid (arrows).

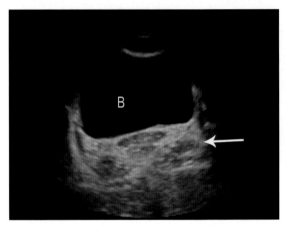

Bladder: Dilated, fluid filled bladder (B) with posterior acoustic enhancement as a result of the low attenuation of the urine (arrow).

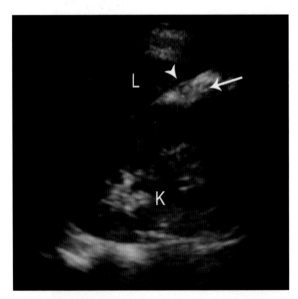

FAST scan of handlebar injury: Perihepatic view. Liver (L), kidney (K), perirenal fat (arrow), small amount of free fluid in hepatorenal space (arrowhead).

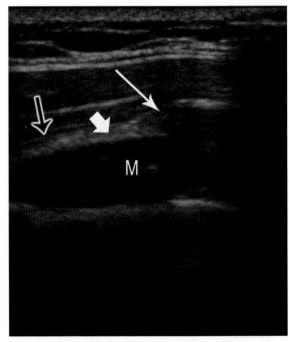

Fractured bone prior to reduction: Fracture site (skinny arrow), medullary cavity (M), cortical bone (fat arrow), periosteum (outlined arrow).

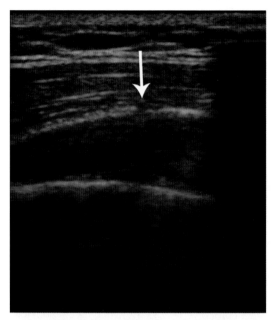

Bone fracture after reduction: Reduced fracture site (arrow).

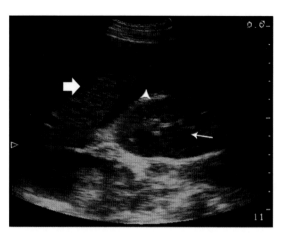

Morrison's pouch: Free fluid within Morrison's pouch between liver and kidney (arrowhead). Liver (fat arrow), kidney (skinny arrow).

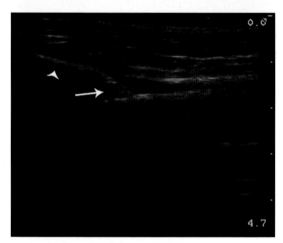

Greenstick fracture: A 6-year-old female with left radius greenstick fracture (arrow). Radius (arrowhead).

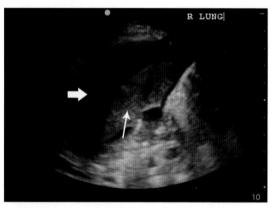

Post-operative complication: Post-operative complication of diaphragm laceration and hemothorax after liver transplant. Transabdominal view of RUQ showing the hemothorax (fat arrow) and lung floating within the hemothorax (skinny arrow).

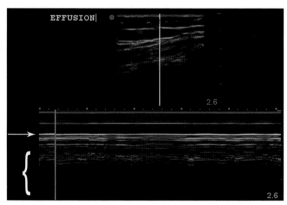

Pleural effusion: M-mode showing characteristic pattern of a pleural effusion. Pleural line (arrow). Note that the granular layer that normally represents respiration movements of the lung is absent (bracket). Normal "seashore sign" is absent.

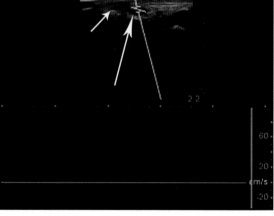

Humerus fracture: Severe left humerus fracture with injury to radial artery. Failure to acquire waveform with Doppler. Radial artery (long arrow), radial vein (short arrow).

Urinary tract

Ultrasound can be used to evaluate the urinary tracts of pediatric patients, including cystitis, obstructive uropathies with enlarged ureters, and hydronephrosis.

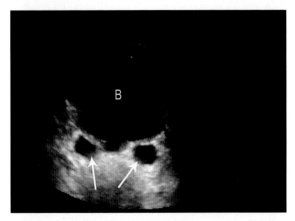

Patient with obstructive uropathy: Transverse view of bladder (B) and bilaterally dilated ureters (arrows).

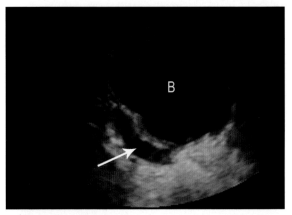

Patient with obstructive uropathy: Sagittal view of bladder (B) with dilated hydroureter (arrow).

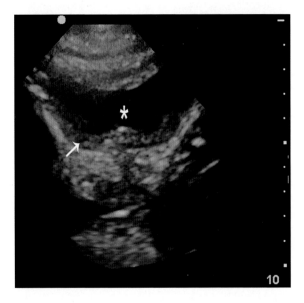

Patient with cystitis: Bladder lumen (asterisk, thickened bladder wall (arrow).

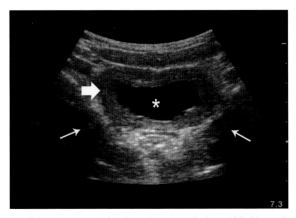

Cystitis: A 6-year-old female with cystitis. Thickened bladder wall (fat arrow), psoas muscle (skinny arrow), bladder lumen (asterisk).

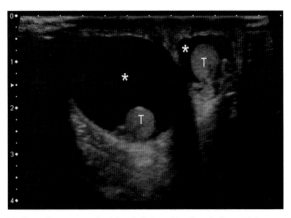

Hydrocele: A 1-week-old with bilateral hydrocele (asterisks), testicles (T's).

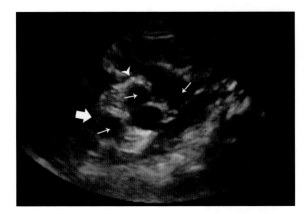

Bilateral hydronephrosis: Left kidney. Dilated renal calyces (arrows), renal cortex (fat arrow), renal capsule (arrowhead).

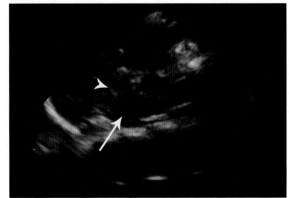

Child with obstructive uropathy and bilateral hydronephrosis: View of right kidney. Dilated renal calyx (arrow), renal cortex (arrowhead).

157

Ultrasound-guided procedures

Eric J. Chin

Ultrasound-guided nerve blocks

Nerve blocks are an ideal way to provide regional anesthesia for patients undergoing painful procedures or with painful conditions. Traditionally, nerve blocks were performed primarily using a landmarks-based approach. Ultrasound is being increasingly utilized with traditional landmarks to provide more accurate anatomical information not previously available and real-time visualization of the nerve being anesthetized.

Axillary block

The axillary block is a relatively safe way to block the distal portion of the brachial plexus to provide anesthesia distal to the elbow region.

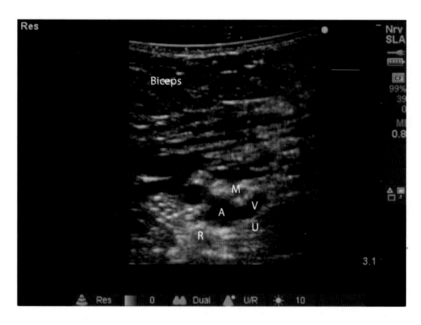

Axillary block, prior to infiltration with anesthetic: The probe should be placed in the axillary region in the transverse plane. In this view, the axillary artery (A) and vein (V) are readily identifiable. The median (M), radial (R), and ulnar (U) nerves will typically be localized around the axillary artery in variable locations.

Atlas of Emergency Ultrasound, ed. John Christian Fox. Published by Cambridge University Press. © J.C. Fox 2011.

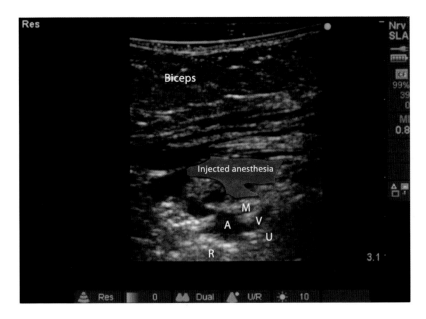

Axillary block, after infiltration with anesthetic: The anesthetic should be injected adjacent to each of the nerves (median (M), radial (R), ulnar (U)) to provide anesthesia for the hand and forearm. The axillary block is generally considered safer than a more proximal brachial plexus approach, however, the musculocutaneous nerve is frequently missed with this technique.

Brachial plexus nerve block

The brachial plexus nerve block is an effective way to provide anesthesia to the entire arm distal to the shoulder region. It can be technically more challenging since the approach is more prone to cause a pneumothorax or vascular insult.

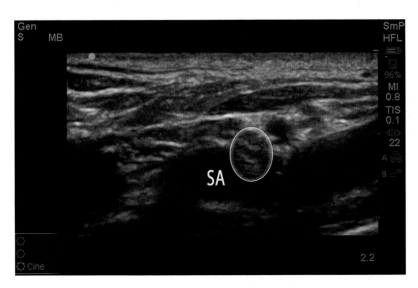

Brachial plexus nerve block, supraclavicular approach: The supraclavicular approach to the brachial plexus nerve block is an effective technique to provide anesthesia to the upper extremity distal to the shoulder. The probe is placed above the middle third of the clavicle angled toward the ipsilateral scapula. In this view, you will see the subclavian artery (SA), and adjacent to it the brachial plexus (circle), which classically has a honeycombed appearance.

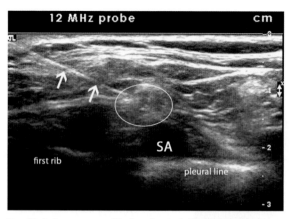

Brachial plexus nerve block prior to infiltration with anesthetic: The needle (arrows) is inserted laterally and directed toward the brachial plexus (circle) and subclavian artery (SA). To avoid an iatrogenic pneumothorax, it is recommended the needle tip be followed during its insertion.

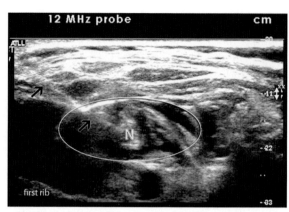

Brachial plexus nerve block after infiltration with anesthetic: Once the needle (arrows) tip approaches the brachial plexus, approximately 25 mL of local anesthetic is injected with real-time visualization of anesthesia (circle) spreading around the brachial plexus (N).

Femoral nerve block

The femoral nerve block is a relatively simple technique that can be used to provided anesthesia to the hip, knee, and anterior thigh.

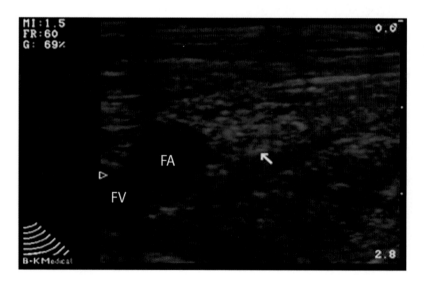

Femoral nerve block anatomy: The probe is placed transversely across the femoral triangle, where you should see the femoral nerve (arrow), femoral artery (FA), and femoral vein (FV).

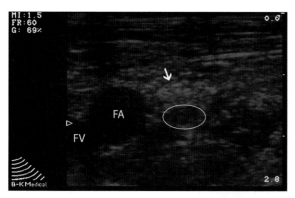

Femoral nerve block during infiltration: The anesthesia (circle) needs to infiltrate deep to the fascia lata (not seen) to ensure the femoral nerve (arrow) is surrounded by local anesthetic. Failure to surround the nerve completely may result in inadequate anesthesia.

Femoral nerve block after infiltration with anesthetic: The anesthesia (outline) can be seen surrounding the femoral nerve (FN), which rests lateral to the femoral artery (FA) and femoral vein (FV).

Median nerve block

The median nerve block is a simple way to provide anesthesia to the first through fourth fingers and lateral portion of the hand.

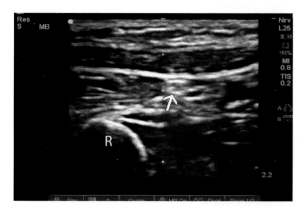

Median nerve block, forearm approach: The median nerve (arrow) should appear as a heteroechoic honey-combed shaped structure within the carpal tunnel or interposed within the forearm flexors, depending on the placement of the ultrasound probe along the forearm. Radius (R).

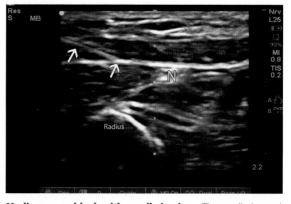

Median nerve block with needle in view: The needle (arrows) can be seen approaching the median nerve (N).

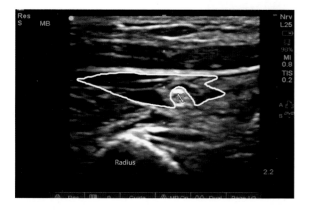

Median nerve block after infiltration of anesthetic: The local anesthesia (outline) is infiltrated around the median nerve (N).

Radial nerve block

The radial nerve block can be used to provide anesthesia to the dorsolateral portions of the hand.

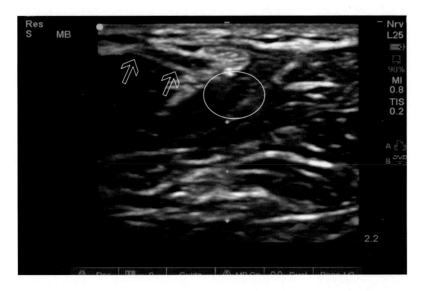

Radial nerve block, forearm approach: The radial nerve (outline) can be located by following its course proximally from the wrist along the radial artery. In this view, the needle can be seen approaching the radial nerve prior to infiltration of a local anesthetic.

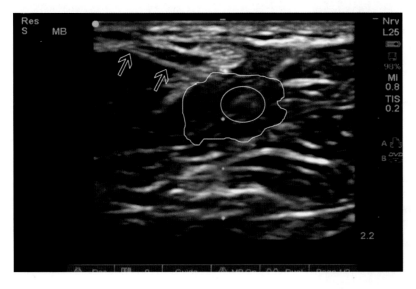

Radial nerve block after infiltration of anesthetic: In this view, the needle (arrows) is seen injecting local anesthesia (outline) around the radial nerve (circle).

Ulnar nerve block

The ulnar nerve block can be utilized to provide anesthesia to the fourth through fifth fingers and medial portion of the hand.

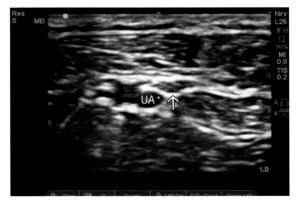

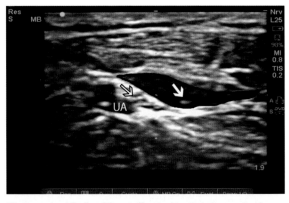

Ulnar nerve block, forearm approach: The ulnar nerve (arrow) can be located anywhere between the wrist and just proximal to the elbow. In this view, the ulnar nerve is located near the ulnar artery (UA).

Ulnar nerve block with needle: In this view, the needle tip (white arrow) can be seen depositing local anesthesia (black outline) next to the ulnar nerve (outlined arrow). Ulnar artery (UA).

Ulnar nerve block after infiltration of anesthetic: Local anesthesia (outline), ulnar nerve (arrow), ulnar artery (UA).

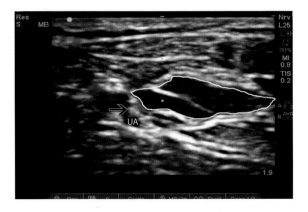

Ultrasound-guided vascular access

Vascular access is a necessity in nearly every aspect of medicine, however, it can be difficult to accomplish in many patients due to a variety of reasons. Ultrasound has been shown to be effective in shortening the time to obtain vascular access, as well as minimizing many of the complications associated with it.

Peripheral IV placement

Ultrasound can be used to facilitate the placement of peripheral IV catheters in patients in whom IV access is difficult to accomplish through standard techniques. It is an effective alternative to more invasive methods of venous access, such as a PICC line and central venous catheter.

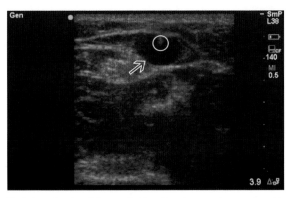

Peripheral vein with needle tip: The ultrasound can assist with localizing superficial or deep peripheral veins (arrow) that are too difficult to palpate. The peripheral vein should be easily compressible to ensure it is not an artery. Needle tip (circle).

163

Internal jugular (IJ) vein central line placement

Ultrasound-guided IJ vein central line placement can be an effective adjunct to expedite the placement of central venous catheters, as well as reducing complications associated with their placement (i.e., pneumothorax, arterial puncture).

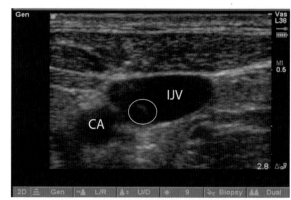

IJ vein after insertion of needle lumen into vessel: IJ vein (IJV), carotid artery (CA), catheter (circle).

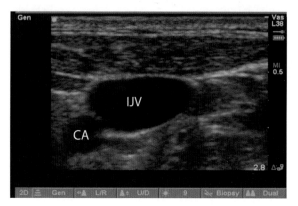

IJ vein anatomy: The IJ vein (IJV) is readily found near the apex of the triangle created by the two heads of the sternocleidomastoid muscle, and is typically located lateral to the carotid artery (CA). The IJ vein is usually easily compressible and its diameter can be augmented by placing the patient in a Trendelenburg position.

Subclavian vein central line placement

Subclavian vein central line placement is traditionally considered to be a blind procedure. With the proper probe placement, ultrasound-guided IJ vein central line placement can be an effective adjunct to expedite the placement of central venous catheters, as well as reducing complications associated with their placement (i.e., pneumothorax, arterial puncture).

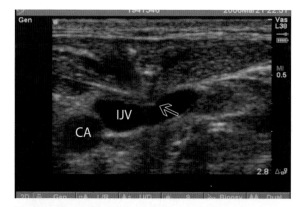

IJ vein with needle tenting blood vessel: Often when attempting to puncture the IJ vein (IJV), the needle tip (arrow) will cause tenting without entering the lumen of the vessel. To ease the entry of the needle tip into the vessel, a very small quick jab with the needle may be enough to get the tip into the vessel. Carotid artery (CA).

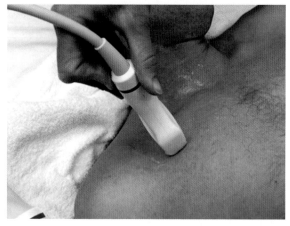

Placement of ultrasound probe for subclavian vein line placement: The probe should be placed inferior to the middle third of the clavicle with the indicator pointing cephalad.

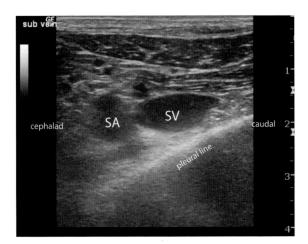

Subclavian vein anatomy: With the probe indicator oriented cephalad, the clavicle (not seen) may be visible on the left side of the image. The subclavian artery (SA) will usually be superior and deep to the subclavian vein (SV). Note the close proximity of the pleural line to the subclavian vein.

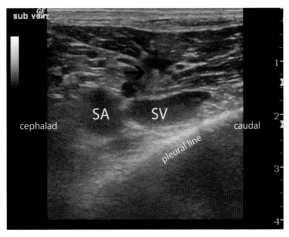

Subclavian vein with needle and tenting of the blood vessel: The distal shaft of the needle (arrow) can be seen tenting the subclavian vein (SV). Subclavian artery (SA).

Subclavian vein with needle in lumen: Subclavian vein (SV) with needle (arrow) in lumen of blood vessel.

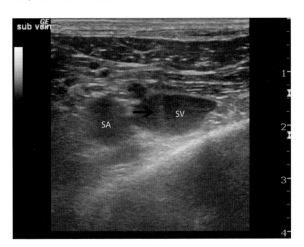

Radial artery line placement

The radial artery line can be a frustrating procedure to perform in the critically ill patient. However, ultrasound-guided radial artery line placement can make it less difficult to localize the radial artery, especially in the hypotensive patient.

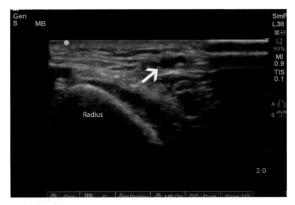

Radial artery anatomy: The ultrasound probe is positioned transversely just proximal to the wrist. The radial artery (arrow) is usually readily seen near the distal radius.

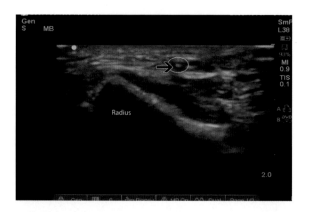

Radial artery line placement: Radial artery line placement with needle (arrow) within lumen or radial artery (circle).

Cardiothoracic procedures
Pericardiocentesis

The pericardiocentesis is a potentially life-saving procedure performed when cardiac tamponade is suspected or recognized in a symptomatic patient. With the use of bedside ultrasound, it is possible to confirm a provider's clinical suspicion for cardiac tamponade and aid in the success of a pericardiocentesis.

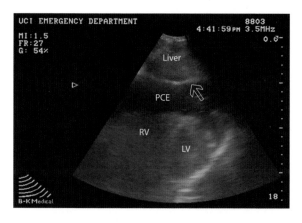

Subxiphoid view of a pericardial effusion: The ultrasound probe is placed just inferior to the xiphoid process and directed cephalad. In this view, the pericardial sac (arrow) can be seen superficial to a pericardial effusion (PCE) that surrounds the right (RV) and left ventricles (LV).

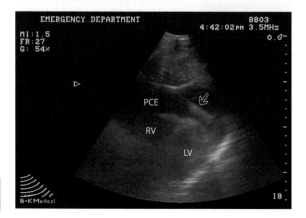

Pericardiocentesis with needle in pericardial space: Traditionally, pericardiocentesis is performed by inserting a needle (arrow) next to the xiphoid process oriented toward the left shoulder. Using ultrasound, it is also possible to aspirate a pericardial effusion (PCE) from a parasternal or apical approach. Right ventricle (RV), left ventricle (LV).

Thoracentesis

A thoracentesis is typically performed by localizing the top of the pleural effusion with percussion to the thoracic cavity. Ultrasound can be used to aid the practitioner performing a thoracentesis in localizing the largest pocket of pleural fluid and minimize the chances of inadvertently puncturing solid organs.

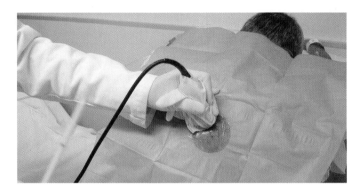

Placement of ultrasound probe for thoracentesis: The ultrasound probe is typically placed posteriorly with the patient in the upright position.

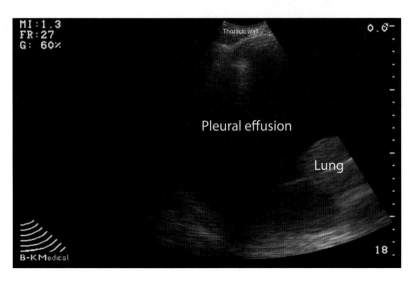

Insertion of thoracentesis needle: The thoracentesis needle should be inserted on the superior side of the rib to minimize the chance of injuring the neurovascular bundle on the inferior side of the rib.

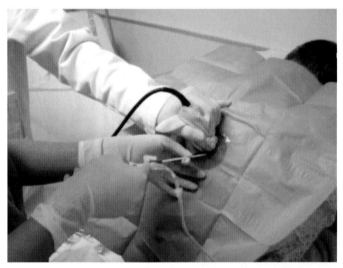

Pleural effusion: You should try to identify the largest fluid pocket, while taking note of the location of the lung and diaphragm (not seen).

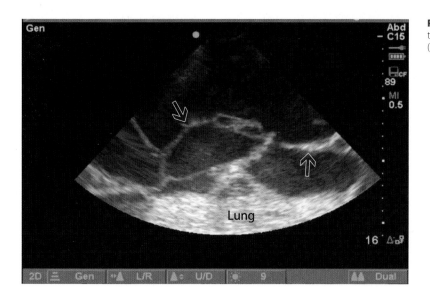

Pleural effusion with loculations: In this view, note the multiple septations (arrows) within the pleural effusion.

Transvenous pacer

Transvenous pacemaker wire placement can be a challenging skill to perform. Ultrasound can be utilized to monitor the real-time placement of the pacing wire lead, thereby improving the likelihood of proper placement.

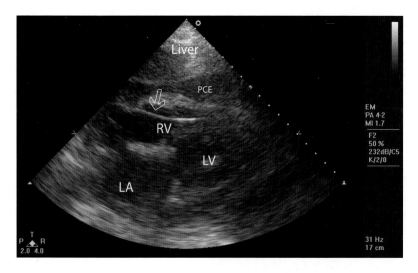

Transvenous pacemaker wire in right ventricle: In this subxiphoid view of the heart, the pacemaker wire (arrow) can be seen entering the right ventricle (RV). Of note, there is also a pericardial effusion (PCE) that can be seen superficial to the heart. Left atrium (LA), left ventricle (LV).

Miscellaneous procedures
Foley balloon rupture

On rare occasions, a Foley catheter can malfunction, with the balloon failing to deflate.

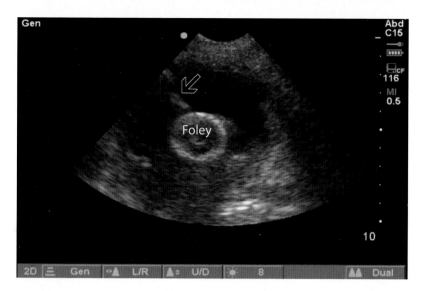

Foley balloon with needle (arrow) in bladder: A malfunctioning Foley balloon can be ruptured by inserting a needle into the bladder suprapubically.

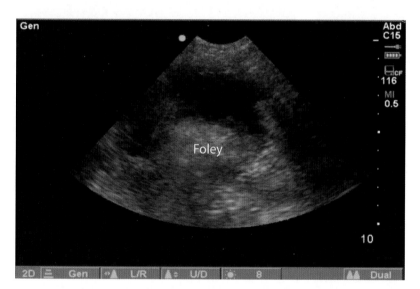

Foley balloon exploding: Foley balloon exploding after puncture with needle.

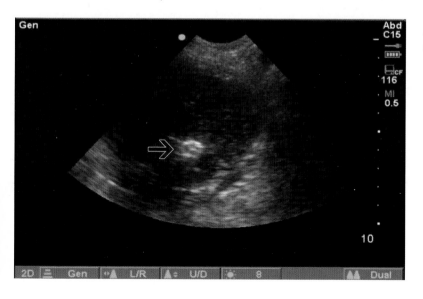

Foley exploded with remaining tube: Residual Foley catheter (arrow) after being ruptured with needle.

Foreign body removal

Foreign bodies can be detected with plain radiographs to varying degrees of success. Ultrasound can be used as a primary or secondary tool to localize foreign bodies within soft tissue. More importantly, ultrasound can be used in real-time to assist with localization of the foreign body and to help minimize damage to surrounding structures.

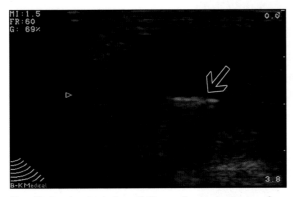

Metallic foreign body in soft tissue: Foreign bodies in soft tissue (arrow) that are difficult to visualize with traditional radiographs may be readily identifiable with ultrasound.

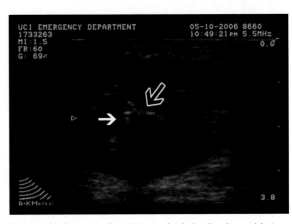

Foreign body extraction: Foreign body (outlined arrow) being extracted from soft tissue with forceps (solid arrow).

Lumbar puncture

The lumbar puncture typically requires the practitioner to readily identify specific landmarks (i.e., the L4-L5 interspinous space) to ensure the successful completion of the procedure. On occasion, it can be nearly impossible to identify the traditional landmarks for the lumbar puncture due to excessive adipose tissue and variations in individual anatomy. Ultrasound can be used to identify the L4-L5 interspinous space, when traditional methods fail to identify the proper landmarks.

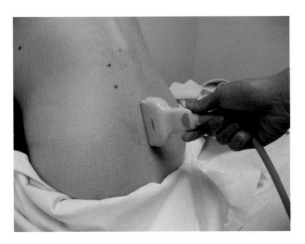

Ultrasound-guided lumbar puncture probe placement, longitudinal plane: Place the probe on the lumbar region midline between an imaginary line across the superior portion of the iliac crests. The indicator should be oriented toward the head.

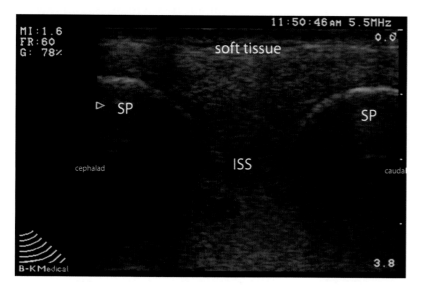

Longitudinal view of spinous processes: After applying the ultrasound probe in the longitudinal axis, move the probe side-to-side and identify the spinous processes (SP), which will appear as hyperechoic curved outlines with shadowing. Then, center the interspinous space (ISS) on the middle of your screen.

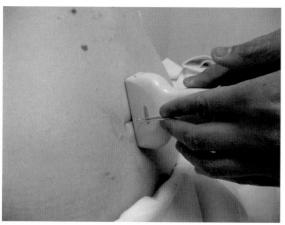

Ultrasound-guided lumbar puncture, horizontal marking: After centering your probe on the interspinous space, you will slide a paperclip under the middle of the probe and hold it in place while you remove the probe from the skin. Using a marker or pen, make a straight line across the paperclip leaving a horizontal mark on the skin.

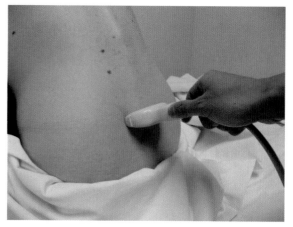

Ultrasound-guided lumbar puncture probe placement, transverse place: Next, you will rotate the probe 90 degrees so that the indicator is toward the left.

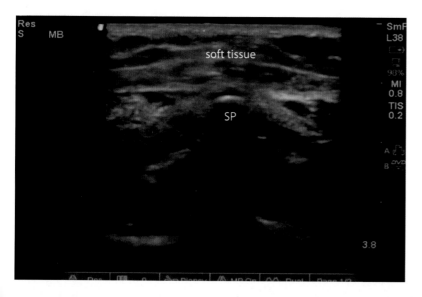

Transverse view of spinous: Move the probe up and down until you are able to identify the spinous process (SP) and move it to the middle of the screen.

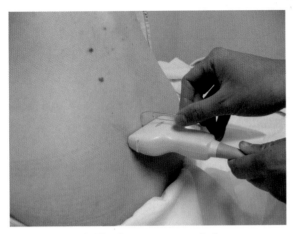

Ultrasound-guided lumbar puncture vertical marking: Again, slide a paperclip under the middle of the probe and hold it in place while you remove the probe from the skin. Using a marker or pen, make another straight line across the paperclip leaving a vertical mark on the skin.

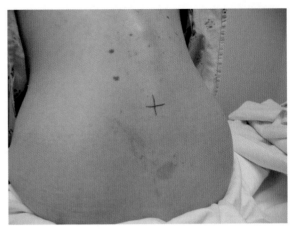

Ultrasound-guided lumbar puncture mark: Using ultrasound to identify your anatomical landmarks for a lumbar puncture should result in a mark at the L4-L5 interspinous space.

Paracentesis

The paracentesis is a relatively safe and easy procedure to perform when there is a large amount of ascites to drain. However, every practitioner will encounter a situation where it is difficult to identify the ideal location to perform the paracentesis. Ultrasound can assist the practitioner to localize the largest pocket of fluid, and thereby minimize the chances of iatrogenic complications.

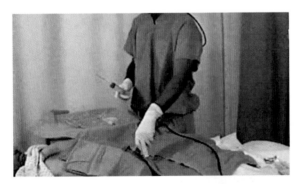

Paracentesis probe placement: To assist with paracentesis, the ultrasound probe can be placed in the traditional locations below the umbilicus or slightly medial and cephalad to the anterior superior iliac spine. However, with real-time visualization it is more practical to use the ultrasound to find the largest fluid pocket away from intra-abdominal structures, such as bowel.

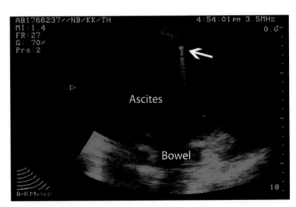

Paracentesis: Paracentesis with large ascites and needle tip (arrow).

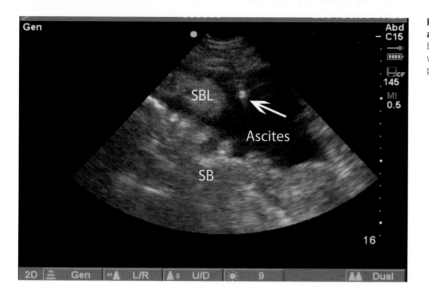

Paracentesis with small bowel loop and needle tip: A loop of small bowel (SBL) can be seen floating in ascites with the needle tip (arrow) inside the peritoneum.

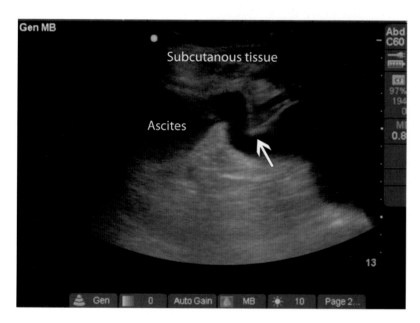

Paracentesis with needle stuck: In this view, a paracentesis is being performed, but the operator is having difficulty getting the needle tip (arrow) to enter the peritoneum.

Peritonsillar abscess drainage

The diagnosis of a peritonsillar abscess is typically made through physical examination and/or computed tomography. Ultrasound can be utilized in combination with the physical examination to identify peritonsillar abscesses without the use of ionizing radiation.

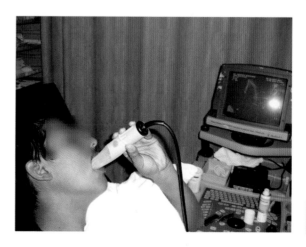

Placement of ultrasound probe for peritonsillar abscess (PTA): The endocavitary probe can be used to distinguish between peritonsillar cellulitis and a peritonsillar abscess. The key to evaluating for a PTA is to anesthetize the posterior pharynx with topical anesthetic, cover the probe with a sheath, and ask the patient to assist in localizing the area of maximal pain with the transducer.

173

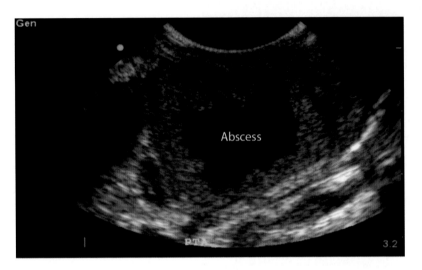

Large peritonsillar abscess, prior to drainage: Peritonsillar abscesses will usually appear hypoechoic and are usually in close proximity to tonsillar tissue.

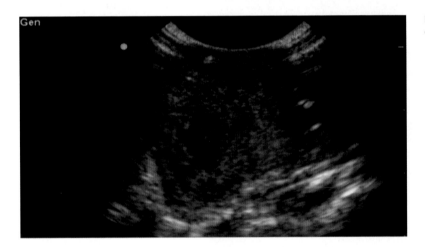

Large peritonsillar abscess, after drainage: This is the same large peritonsillar abscess after aspiration with a needle.

Cellulitis

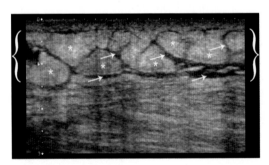

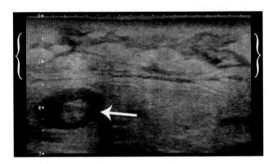

Cellulitis: Cellulitis in right calf with "cobblestoning" ("{}"). Hyperechoic subcutaneous tissue (asterisks) with subcutaneous edema filling the interlobar septae (arrows).

Cellulitis: Cellulitis ("{}"), lymph node (arrow).

Arterial ultrasound

Sharis Simonian and John Christian Fox

Carotid artery stenosis

Carotid artery stenosis is typically diagnosed and assessed with a color flow duplex ultrasound scan of the carotid arteries in the neck. Carotid artery stenosis can manifest itself as asymptomatic or symptomatic. Generally, carotid artery duplex ultrasound scans are a safe and relatively inexpensive method for evaluation of carotid artery stenosis.

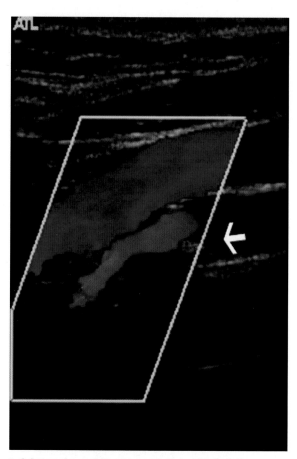

Left internal carotid artery stenosis, sagittal view, > 70%: Sagittal view of a proximal left internal carotid artery demonstrating greater than 70% stenosis. The white arrow demonstrates abnormal artery intima secondary to plaque.

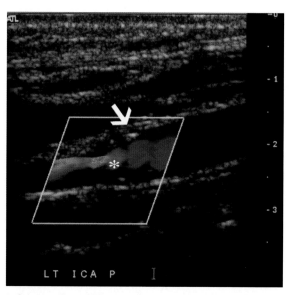

Left internal carotid artery stenosis, > 70%: A 71-year-old male with proximal left internal carotid artery displaying greater than 70% stenosis, demonstrated in Doppler flow. The white arrow indicates abnormal carotid artery intima. The white asterisk demonstrates the lumen of the artery.

Atlas of Emergency Ultrasound, ed. John Christian Fox. Published by Cambridge University Press. © J.C. Fox 2011.

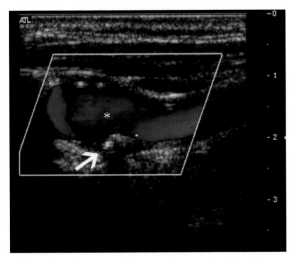

Left common carotid artery bulb stenosis, with color Doppler: Left common carotid artery bulb demonstrated with color Doppler flow, indicating an occlusion with greater than 50% stenosis of the bulb. The white arrow demonstrates the plaque leading to an abnormal carotid artery intima. The white asterisk indicates the lumen of the carotid artery.

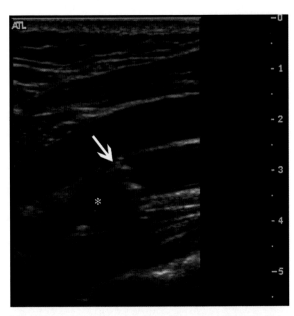

Left common carotid artery bulb stenosis, > 70%: Sagittal view of the left common carotid artery bulb, demonstrating significant stenosis. White arrow indicates plaque leading to an abnormal carotid artery intima. White asterisk demonstrates lumen of the artery.

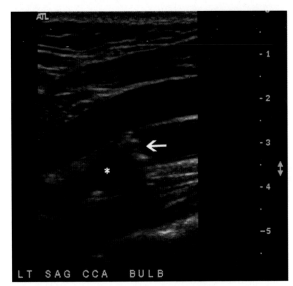

Left common carotid artery (CCA) bulb stenosis, > 70%: Sagittal view of the left common carotid artery bulb. The white arrow indicates plaque within the CCA bulb, with greater than 70% stenosis. The white asterisk indicates the lumen of the artery.

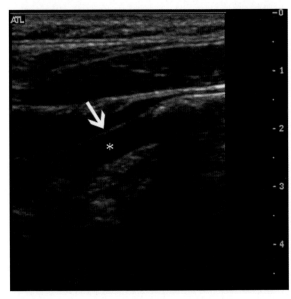

Proximal left external carotid artery, no occlusion: Proximal left external carotid artery, with no evidence of occlusion of blood flow. White arrow demonstrates normal intima. White asterisk points to lumen of artery.

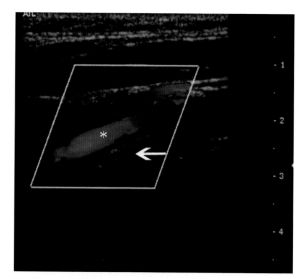

Proximal left external carotid artery, no occlusion: Proximal left external carotid artery, with color Doppler flow. White arrow indicates normal carotid intima. White asterisk indicates lumen of carotid artery.

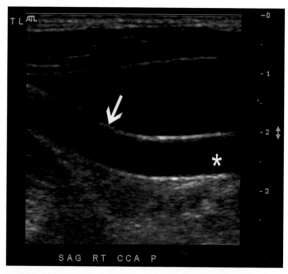

Right common carotid artery, sagittal view, normal intima: Sagittal view of right common carotid artery, demonstrating normal intimal thickness (arrow). Asterisk indicates lumen of carotid artery.

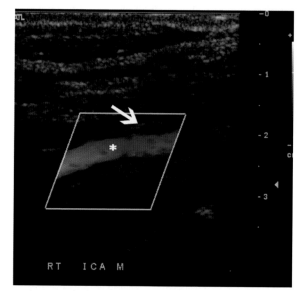

Right internal carotid artery, sagittal view, normal intima: Right internal carotid artery with color Doppler imaging. The white arrow indicates normal carotid artery intima. Asterisk demonstrates lumen of artery.

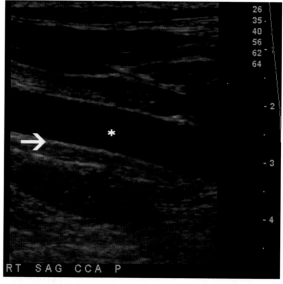

Right common carotid artery, sagittal view, normal intima: Sagittal view of proximal right common carotid artery. The white arrow demonstrates normal carotid intima. The white asterisk indicates the lumen of the artery.

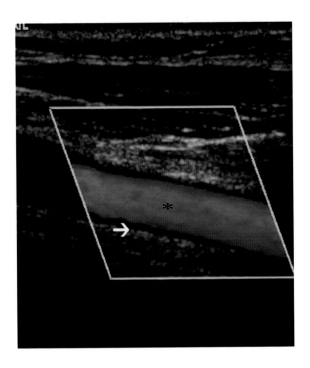

Right common carotid artery, sagittal view, normal intima: Sagittal view of right common carotid artery, with Doppler flow. The white arrow demonstrates normal carotid artery intima. The black asterisk indicates arterial lumen.

Abdominal aortic aneurysm

The traditional abdominal aortic aneurysm (AAA) triad demonstrates with hypotension, pulsatile abdominal mass, and back pain. Ultrasound is a reliable modality for initial screening and diagnosis of an abdominal aortic aneurysm. Generally, surgical repair is indicated for AAA diameters exceeding 5.5 cm in males and 5.0 cm in females.

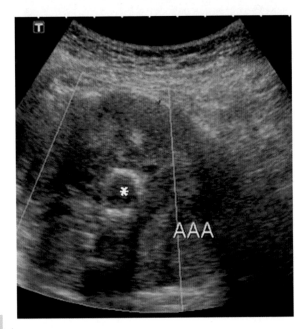

Abdominal aortic aneurysm, transverse view: Transverse view of the abdominal aortic aneurysm (AAA). The green line outlines the AAA. The white asterisk demonstrates the lumen of the abdominal aorta.

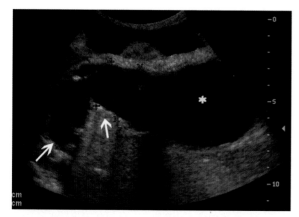

Abdominal aortic fusiform aneurysm, sagittal view: Sagittal view of distal abdominal aortic fusiform aneurysm. The white arrow demonstrates the fusiform shape of the aneurysm. The yellow asterisk points out the lumen of the abdominal aorta proper.

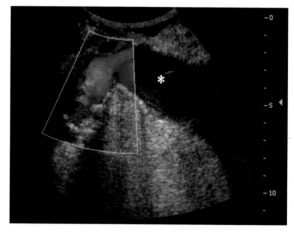

Abdominal aortic fusiform aneurysm, demonstrated with color Doppler: Abdominal aortic fusiform aneurysm, with color Doppler ultrasound. The green line outlines the fusiform aneurysm portion of the abdominal aorta. The white asterisk indicates the lumen of the abdominal aorta proper.

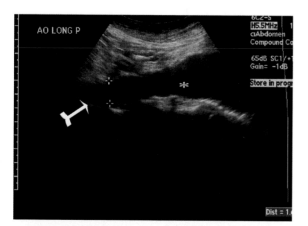

Fusiform abdominal aortic aneurysm: An 80-year-old female demonstrating fusiform abdominal aortic aneurysm. The white arrow points out the fusiform appearance of the aneurysm. The yellow asterisk indicates the lumen of the abdominal aorta.

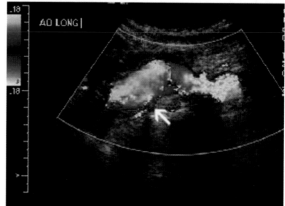

Fusiform abdominal aortic aneurysm, sagittal view: Sagittal view of a color Doppler ultrasound image of a 76-year-old female with a fusiform abdominal aortic aneurysm. White arrow points out fusiform aneurysm.

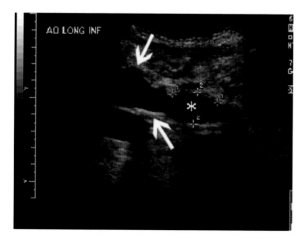

Fusiform abdominal aortic aneurysm: Sagittal view of abdominal aorta fusiform aneurysm. White arrows demonstrate fusiform aneurysm. White asterisk indicates the lumen of the aorta.

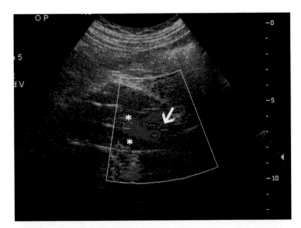

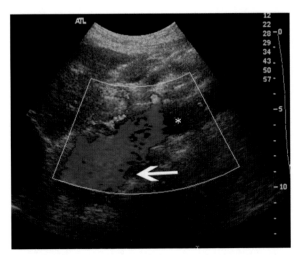

Abdominal aortic aneurysm and patent graft, sagittal view, demonstrated in color Doppler: Sagittal view of abdominal aortic aneurysm with patent graft in color Doppler. White arrow demonstrates the patent graft within the aorta. The two white asterisks indicate the two lumens of the aorta status post graft placement.

Abdominal aortic aneurysm and patent graft, sagittal view, demonstrated in color Doppler: Sagittal view of the abdominal aortic aneurysm (AAA), with color Doppler ultrasound. White arrow demonstrates aneurysm. White asterisk points out lumen of the aorta.

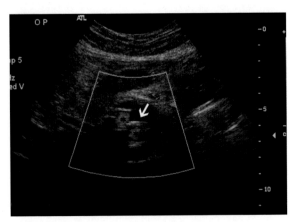

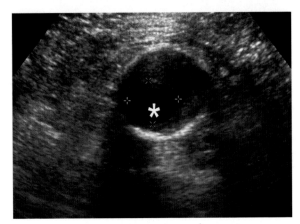

Abdominal aortic aneurysm and patent graft, transverse view, demonstrated in color Doppler: Transverse view of the abdominal aortic aneurysm with patent graft in color Doppler. The white arrow demonstrates the patent graft. The two black asterisks indicate the two abdominal aortic lumens present status post graft placement.

Abdominal aortic aneurysm, with large thrombus: Abdominal aortic aneurysm with large thrombus occluding the lumen. Asterisk indicates non-occluded portion of the lumen.

Abdominal aortic aneurysm and patent graft, transverse view: Transverse view of the abdominal aortic aneurysm with patent graft in place. White arrow demonstrates the patent graft within the aorta. The two white asterisks indicate the abdominal aorta status post graft placement.

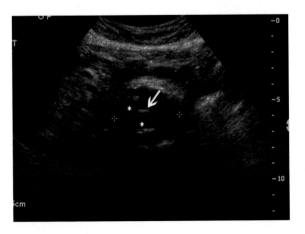

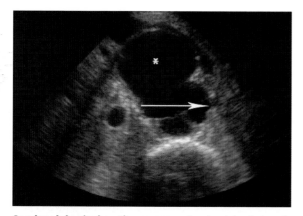

Sacular abdominal aortic aneurysm: Sacular abdominal aortic aneurysm. The white arrow demonstrates the width of the sacular aneurysm. The yellow asterisk indicates the lumen of the proper abdominal aorta.

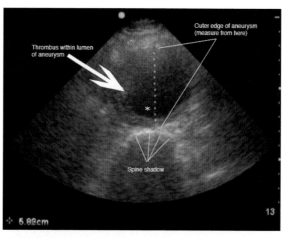

Abdominal aortic aneurysm, with thrombus: Abdominal aortic aneurysm with significant thrombus. White arrow demonstrates the mural thrombus. The dotted white line measures the outer edge of the abdominal aneurysm. The yellow lines indicate the spine shadow. White asterisk points out lumen of aorta.

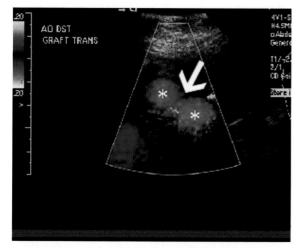

Abdominal aortic aneurysm, with patent graft, transverse view: Transverse view of a distal abdominal aorta with evidence of patent graft, in color Doppler flow. White arrow indicates the patent graft. The two white asterisks point out the lumens of the iliacs.

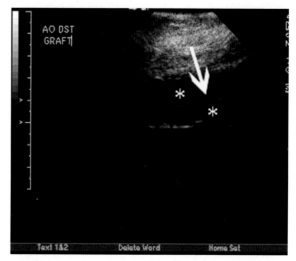

Abdominal aortic aneurysm, with patent graft, sagittal view: Transverse view of distal abdominal aorta, with patent graft. White arrow indicates region of the graft. White asterisks point out the two lumens of the aorta.

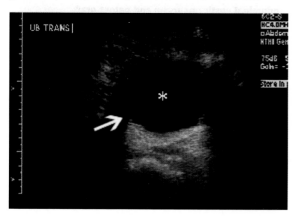

Abdominal aortic aneurysm: This is an example of an abdominal aortic aneurysm that measures 5.5 cm.

Femoral artery pseudoaneurysm

Femoral artery pseudoaneurysm is a common complication of cardiac catheterizations. A femoral artery pseudoaneurysm often manifests as a pulsatile mass with a systolic bruit overlying the insertion site. Ultrasound duplex imaging can confirm the presence of a femoral artery pseudoaneurysm.

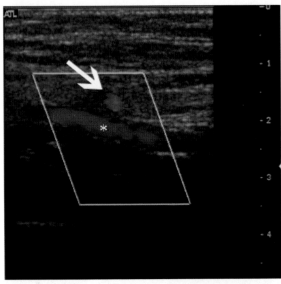

Right common femoral artery pseudoaneurysm: Right common femoral artery pseudoaneurysm, status post cardiac catheterization, with color Doppler imaging. White arrow demonstrates portion of artery that is considered the pseudoaneurysm. White asterisk indicates lumen of the artery.

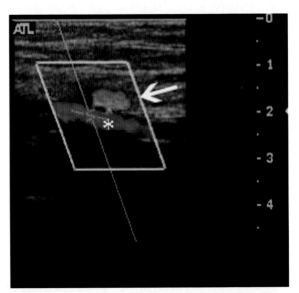

Right common femoral artery pseudoaneurysm: Color Doppler ultrasound image of right femoral artery pseudoaneurysm. White arrow points out pseudoaneurysm. White asterisk displays lumen of artery proper.

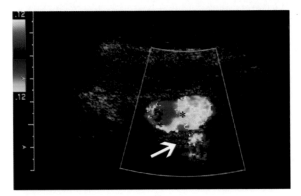

Right common femoral artery pseudoaneurysm: Color Doppler ultrasound image of right femoral artery pseudoaneurysm status post cardiac catheterization. White arrow demonstrates pseudoaneurysm portion of the artery. Black asterisk indicates lumen of the femoral artery.

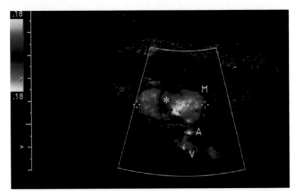

Right femoral artery pseudoaneurysm, with color Doppler flow: Color Doppler ultrasound transverse image of a pseudoaneurysm of the right femoral artery. White "V" indicates femoral vein. White asterisk lumen of femoral artery.

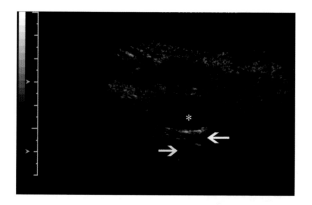

Right femoral artery pseudoaneurysm, transverse view: Transverse view of right femoral artery status post cardiac catheterization. White arrow demonstrates pseudoaneurysm of the artery. Yellow arrow points out femoral vein. White asterisk indicates lumen of femoral artery.

Renal artery embolism

Renal artery embolism is an uncommon, but acute, diagnosis, which may lead to renal artery occlusion and ultimately, renal failure and necrosis. Ultrasound imaging is one of several different imaging modalities utilized to visualize renal artery emboli to renal arteries.

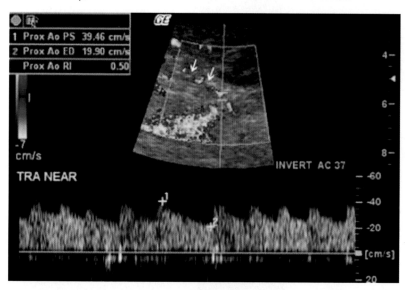

Renal artery embolism: This image depicts a renal artery embolism, which leads to a renal artery infarction. The white arrows in the image indicate the region of infarction, with absence of Doppler flow in the region.

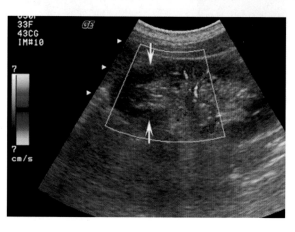

Renal artery embolism: This image depicts renal artery embolism in the intrarenal arteries of the upper pole of the kidney. The white arrows demonstrate absence of color Doppler flow through the upper pole of the kidney due to the embolism.

Renal artery thrombosis

Renal artery thrombosis is an acute diagnosis, which may lead to an acute renal infarct and ultimate renal failure. Ultrasound imaging is a modality used to visualize thrombi and an area of hypoperfusion secondary to a renal artery thrombosis.

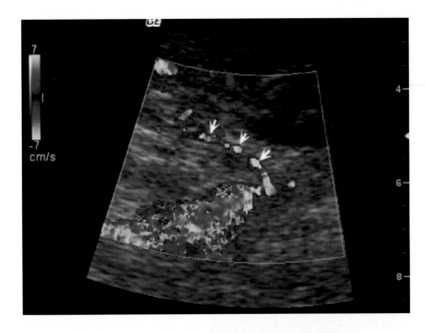

Renal artery thrombosis: This image depicts a partially occlusive renal artery thrombosis. The white arrows depict areas of decreased blood flow via color Doppler imaging.

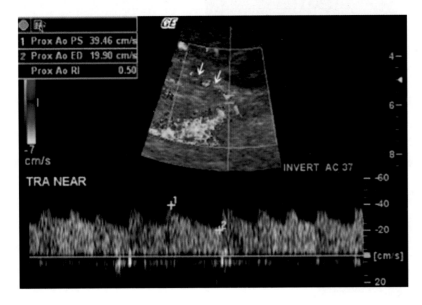

Renal artery thrombosis: This image depicts a transplant renal artery with partially occlusive thrombosis. The white arrows indicate areas of thromboses. The Doppler spectrum depicts the low velocity of flow in the artery.

Chapter 13

Venous ultrasound

Kevin Burns and John Christian Fox

Normal venous anatomy and negative compression testing

The deep veins of the leg are common locations for thrombosis due to immobility or a hypercoagulable state. In a normal patient, the deep veins run with a paired artery and are fully compressible. Compression ultrasonography can be performed along the length of the femoral and popliteal vein at the bedside to quickly rule out deep venous thrombosis (DVT).

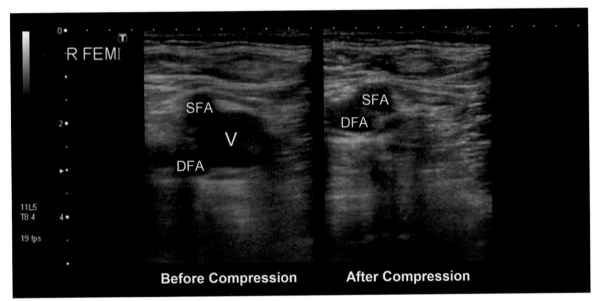

Normal right femoral vein: The transducer is placed transversely to view the right femoral vein (V), superficial femoral artery (SFA) and deep femoral artery (DFA) in cross-section. While visualizing the femoral vein and artery, pressure is applied via the transducer to compress the vein. The femoral vein compresses completely while the arteries remain patent, ruling out venous thrombus at this location.

Atlas of Emergency Ultrasound, ed. John Christian Fox. Published by Cambridge University Press. © J.C. Fox 2011.

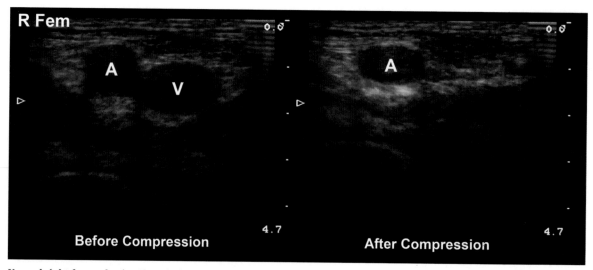

Before Compression   **After Compression**

Normal right femoral vein: The right femoral vein (V) is seen medial to the femoral artery (A). The transducer is used to compress the vein indicating the absence of thrombus. Cycles of compression-decompression are continued along the length of the vein to exclude venous thrombosis.

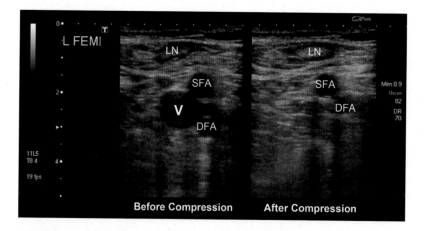

Normal left femoral vein: The left femoral vein (V) is visualized medial to the superficial (SFA) and deep femoral arteries (DFA) along with a superficial lymph node (LN). When the transducer is pressed firmly, the normal vein will collapse and the arteries will remain open.

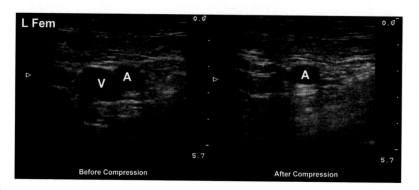

Normal left femoral vein: The transducer is used to visualize the left femoral vein (V) with and without compression. The femoral artery (A) will remain patent when applying cycles of pressure along the vein. Complete collapse of the vein during compression indicates the absence of thrombosis.

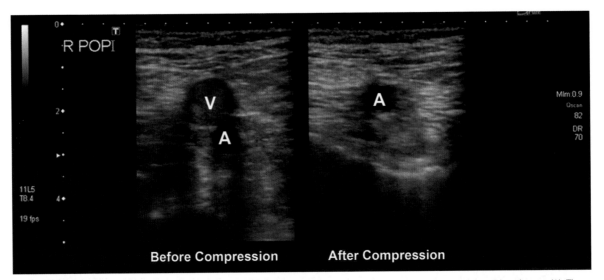

Normal popliteal vein: The transducer is placed transversely in the popliteal fossa to visualize the popliteal vein (V) and artery (A). The popliteal artery is deep to the vein. A patent popliteal vein will compress completely when pressure is applied and the artery may appear more superficial due to compression of the surrounding soft tissue.

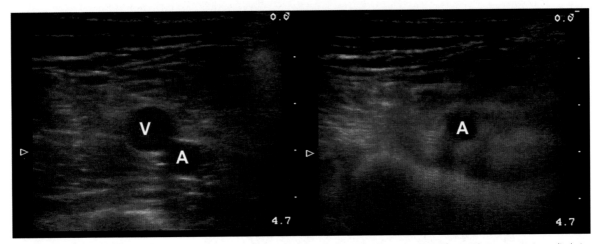

Normal popliteal vein: The popliteal vein (V) and artery (A) are seen in cross-section in the popliteal fossa. When pressure is applied via the transducer, the vein collapses while the artery remains patent.

Deep venous thrombosis (DVT)

In the setting of suspected pulmonary embolism or lower extremity swelling, compression ultrasonography can be used in the emergency department to detect a DVT, allowing the clinician to quickly begin treatment and prevent significant morbidity and mortality from embolization.

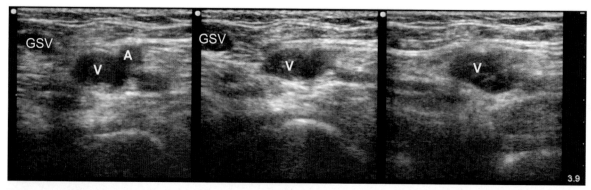

Non-compressible femoral vein thrombosis: There is a thrombus in the left common femoral vein (V) preventing collapse when increasing amounts of pressure are applied. The great saphenous vein (GSV) also contains a thrombus and is non-compressible. The pressure applied to the vessels is great enough to collapse the femoral artery (A). In a normal patient, the vein should compress without compressing the artery. These findings are positive for deep venous thrombosis.

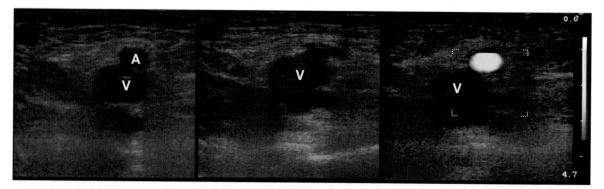

Femoral vein thrombosis: The left common femoral vein (V) contains a non-compressible thrombus. When the transducer is used to compress the vein, the accompanying artery (A) collapses while the vein maintains its shape (2). Color flow Doppler imaging reveals the absence of blood flow in the thrombosed vein (3).

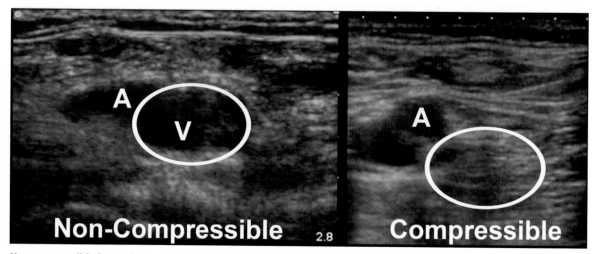

Non-compressible femoral vein with thrombus compared to compressible vein: The right femoral vein is visualized after pressure is applied to the vessels in a patient with a thrombus (left) and normal patient (right). The thrombus prevents the walls of the vein (V) from collapsing, even under enough pressure to deform the appearance of the artery (A).

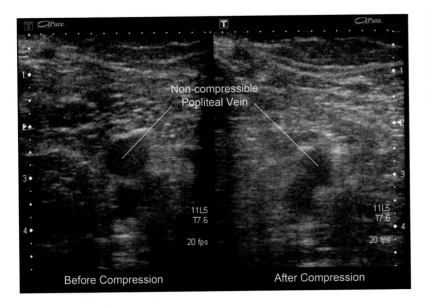

Popliteal vein with thrombosis: A thrombus in the popliteal vein prevents collapse when the transducer is pressed firmly in the popliteal fossa. The popliteal artery is deep to the vein. This finding indicates deep venous thrombosis at the level of the knee.

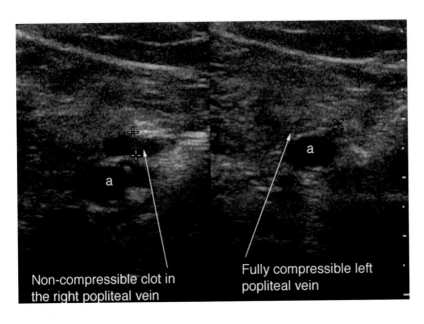

Non-compressible clot in the right popliteal vein compared to fully compressible left popliteal vein: This patient has a thrombus in the right popliteal vein and a patent left popliteal vein. Images of both veins are shown after compression is applied via the transducer. The thrombus prevents collapse of the right popliteal vein, while the normal vein disappears. The popliteal artery (A) remains open.

Upper extremity DVT

Thrombosis in the veins of the upper extremity and neck can occur secondary to central venous or peripherally inserted central catheter placement, transvenous pacemakers, or hypercoagulable states.

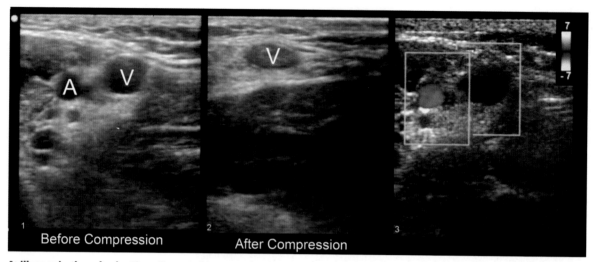

Axillary vein thrombosis: The axillary vein (V) is imaged with the transducer placed in the infraclavicular region with the patient's, arm abducted to 90 degrees. The vein does not compress when enough pressure to collapse the axillary artery (A) is applied using the transducer. No blood movement is seen in the vein using color flow Doppler.

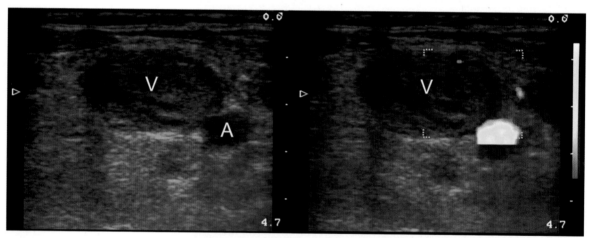

Jugular vein thrombosis: The jugular vein lumen (V) is filled with a non-compressible occlusive thrombus. The vein fails to compress and demonstrates no flow on color flow Doppler imaging.

Index

A-lines, pulmonary 35, 36–7, 38
abdominal aortic aneurysm 178–81
abdominal paracentesis 172–3
abdominal trauma 4–6, 9–13, 154
abscesses
   peritonsillar 147, 173–4
   renal 110
   scrotal 125
   soft tissue 147
   testicular 125
Achilles tendon, ruptured 139
aerobilia 67
air bronchograms 49–51
alveolar interstitial syndrome
   45–8
ankle 133
   effusion 138
aortic aneurysm, abdominal 178–81
aortic dissection, proximal 33
aortic regurgitation 33
aortic valve, bicuspid 32
apical views of heart 27–8
appendicitis 78–82, 141–6
   psoas rectus compression 80–1
   ring of fire 82
appendicolith 141
appendix 77–82
   free fluid around 79
   normal 77
   perforated 79, 144, 145
arterial ultrasound 175–84
ascites 64–5, 82–3
   paracentesis 172–3
   ventral hernias 84, 85
atrial myxoma 34
atrial septal defect 34
axillary nerve block 158–9
axillary vein thrombosis 190

B-lines, pulmonary 45–8
barcode (stratosphere) sign
   40, 42, 43
bat sign 36
BB pellets 150, 151
bee stinger 150
biliary anatomy 58–9
biliary polyps 69–70
biliary sludge 68–9
biloma 69

bladder, urinary 13, 114–17
   masses 115–16
   stones 116
   volume measurement 114
brachial plexus nerve block 159–60
brachial vein 149

cardiac tamponade 29–30, 166
cardiac ultrasound see heart
cardiothoracic procedures 166–8
carotid artery stenosis 175–8
cellulitis 174
central venous line placement 149,
   164–5
cervical lymphadenitis 146
chest trauma 1–4, 6–7, 8–9
cholangiocarcinoma 74
cholelithiasis 59–62
cirrhotic liver 73
common bile duct (CBD) 63–4
compression testing
   appendicitis 80–1, 143, 145, 146
   deep venous thrombosis
     187–9, 190
   negative 185–7
   veins for vascular access 149, 163,
     164
corpus luteal cysts 98, 99
cystic duct 59
cystitis, pediatric 116, 156

deep venous thrombosis (DVT) 187–9
   negative compression testing 185–7
   upper extremity 189–90
diaphragm laceration 155
dilated cardiomyopathy 30
dislocations 135–8
diverticulitis 83–4
double arch (WES) sign 70–1
duodenum 71–2, 83

ectopic pregnancy 90, 93, 94–6
elbow 133, 140
emphysema, subcutaneous 44
empyema, pleural 55
endocarditis, infective 34
epicardial fat pad 1
epididymal cyst 124
epididymitis 128–31

epididymo-orchitis 128, 131
eye 19–25

FAST 1–8, 150
fecaliths
   appendiceal 142–3
   duodenal 72
   intestinal diverticula 84
female patients
   pelvic ultrasound 88–102
   suprapubic FAST 13–14
femoral artery pseudoaneurysm 182–3
femoral fracture 136
femoral nerve block 160–1
femoral vein 186
   thrombosis 188
fibroid uterus 101–2
finger, dislocated 136
focused assessment of sonography in
   trauma (FAST) 1–8, 150
Foley catheter 116
   balloon rupture 168–9
foreign bodies
   pediatric patients 150–1
   rectal 87
   removal 170
fractures 135–8, 154–5

gallbladder 58
   contracted 66
   wall-echo-shadow (WES) sign 70–1
   wall thickening 65–6
gallstones 59–62
genitourinary ultrasound 103–32
globe (of eye), ruptured 19–20
gout 139
great saphenous vein, thrombus 188
gunshot wounds (GSW)
   chest 7, 30
   eye 19
   pediatric patients 150, 151
   testis 120

hand 140
handlebar injury 154
heart 26–34
   enlargement 30–1
   fluid collections around 29–30
   normal views 26–8

heart (cont.)
  strain, right 31–2
  trauma 1–4, 6–7, 150
  valvular dysfunction 32–4
hemangioma, hepatic 74–5
hemopericardium 1–2, 30
hemothorax 8–9, 155
hepatic ducts, dilated 72–3
hernias 84–5
hip 135
  effusion 140
beta-human chorionic gonadotropin
  (hCG) 91, 93, 94, 96
humerus fracture 155
hydrocele 126–7, 130–1, 151, 157
hydronephrosis 110–12, 157
hydroureter 110–12
hypernephroma 107–8
hypertrophic obstructive
  cardiomyopathy (HOCM) 30

infections, pediatric 146–7
infective endocarditis 34
inguinal hernia 84, 121
internal jugular vein 149, 164
intestinal ultrasound 77–87
intracranial pressure, raised 20
intrauterine devices 90, 93
intrauterine pregnancy 91–3
intravenous (IV) access 163–5
  pediatric patients 149
intussusception 85–6, 148–9

joints
  dislocations 135–8
  normal 133–5
  pathology 138–40
jugular vein thrombosis 190

kidney 103–13
  atrophic 105–6
  horseshoe 106
  masses, cysts and abscesses
    106–10
  normal 103–4
  pelvic 106
  variations 105–6
knee 134
  effusion 139

left chest
  FAST 2–4
  fluid in 4
left ventricular aneurysm,
  apical 31
left ventricular hypertrophy 31
leiomyomas, uterine 101–2
ligament pathology 138–40
liver

main lobar fissure 58
metastases 73–4
pathology 72–5
lumbar puncture 170–2
lung 35–57
  alveolar consolidation 49–51
  hepatization 49, 51
  interstitial syndrome 45–8
  mirror-image artifact 52
  white 48
lung point
  false 41, 42
  pneumothorax 41, 42
lung pulse sign 39

male patients
  genital tract 117
  suprapubic FAST 14–18
median nerve block 161
metacarpophalangeal joint 134
metastatic liver disease 73–4
Mickey Mouse sign 58, 70
mirror-image artifact, lung 52
mitral regurgitation 33
mitral stenosis 31
mitral valve prolapse 32
molar pregnancy 96–7
Morrison's pouch 4–6, 155
musculoskeletal ultrasound 133–40

Nabothian cysts 95, 100
nasal fracture 137
nephroblastoma (Wilms' tumor)
  108–9, 151
nerve blocks 158–63

O-lines, pulmonary 39
obstructive uropathy 110–12,
  156, 157
ocular ultrasound 19–25
olecranon bursitis 140
olive sandwich sign 64
optic nerve 20
orchitis 122
ovarian cysts 98–100
  corpus luteal 98, 99
  hemorrhagic 96, 100
  Nabothian 95, 100
  theca lutein 97
ovarian mass 151
ovarian torsion 100–1
ovaries 88, 89

pacemakers, transvenous 168
pancreas 75–6
pancreatic duct of Wirsung 75
paracentesis, abdominal 172–3
parasternal long axis (PLAX) view of
  heart 26

parasternal short axis (PSAX) views of
  heart 27
pediatric ultrasound 141–57
pelvis 88–102
  female anatomy 88–91
  free fluid 6, 90–1, 95–6
  trauma, FAST 4–6, 9–18
penile fractures 132
penile implants 132
pericardial clot 6–7
pericardial effusion 29, 54, 166
pericardial tamponade 29–30, 166
pericardiocentesis 29, 166
perinephric fat 8, 103–4
peripheral intravenous (IV) access
  149, 163
peritonsillar abscess 147
  drainage 173–4
Playboy Bunny sign 59
pleural effusion 52–7
  alveolar consolidation with 51
  liver disease 75
  pediatric patients 147, 155
  thoracentesis 56, 167–8
pneumobilia 67
pneumonia 147
pneumothorax (PTX) 40–4
polycystic kidney disease 112–13
popliteal vein 187
  thrombosis 189
pouch of Douglas, free fluid 90–1
power slide sign 38, 43
pregnancy
  abnormal 89, 93
  ectopic 90, 93, 94–6
  intrauterine 91–3
  molar 96–7
procedures, ultrasound-assisted
  158–74
prostate, enlarged 116–17
psoas rectus compression, appendicitis
  80–1
pulmonary edema 47
pulmonary embolism 31–2
pyloric stenosis 151–3

quad sign 53

radial artery
  injury 155
  line placement 165–6
radial nerve block 162
radius fractures 135, 155
rectal foreign body 87
renal abscess 110
renal artery
  duplicate 106
  embolism 183
  thrombosis 184

renal blood flow 104
renal calculus 109, 112
renal cell carcinoma 107–8
renal cysts 109–10
renal ultrasound 103–13
rete testis, tubular ectasia 125–4
retinal detachment 21–5
right chest, FAST 8–9
right upper quadrant ultrasonography
    58–76
ring of fire
    appendicitis 82
    ectopic pregnancy 94

scaphoid 134
    fracture 137
scrotal abscess 125
scrotal hematoma 120
scrotal hernia *see* inguinal hernia
seashore sign 36, 37, 38, 42
shoulder 133
    dislocation 136, 137
shred sign 51
sinusoid sign 52
skin infections 146, 147
skull fracture 138
sludge, biliary 68–9
small bowel
    obstruction 86
    peristalsis 82

spermatocele 122
spine sign 49, 50
splenic vein 75
splenorenal view, FAST 9–13
stab wounds, chest 2
sternal fracture 138
stratosphere sign 40, 42, 43
subchorionic hemorrhage 93
subclavian vein 164–5
subcutaneous air 44
subxiphoid view of heart 26
superior mesenteric artery 75, 76
suprapubic view, FAST 13–18
suprasternal view of heart 28

testes 117–25
    abscess 125
    blood flow 118
    cyst 124
    fractured 120
    gun shot wound 120
    mass adjacent to 123–4
    microlithiasis 123
    torsion 119
testicular appendix 118, 151
testicular carcinoma 123
theca lutein cysts 97
thoracentesis 56, 167–8
tibial fracture 137
transvenous pacemakers 168

trauma 1–8
    pediatric 150, 154–5

ulnar nerve block 163
ultrasound-assisted procedures
    158–74
umbilical hernia 85
upper extremity deep venous
    thrombosis 189–90
urinary tract 103–17
    pediatric 156–7
uterus 88–9
    bicornuate 89
    fibroid 101–2

valvular heart dysfunction 32–4
varicocele 122
vascular access 149, 163–6
venous ultrasound 185–90
ventral hernia 84, 85
ventricular septal defect 33
vitreous 25

wall-echo-shadow (WES) sign 70–1
water bath 138, 140
white lung 48
Wilms' tumor 108–9, 151
wrist 134

Z-line, lung ultrasound 36